COMMUNICATION
FOR
DENTAL AUXILIARIES

COMMUNICATION FOR DENTAL AUXILIARIES

CHERYL B. WILES M.S., R.D.H.
Dental Hygiene Educator

WILLIAM J. RYAN
Department of Communication
Rockhurst College

RESTON PUBLISHING COMPANY, INC.
A Preston-Hall Company
RESTON, VIRGINIA

Library of Congress Cataloging in Publication Data

Wiles, Cheryl B.
   Communication for dental auxiliaries

   Includes bibliographies and index.
   1. Communication in dentistry.   2. Dental personnel
and patient.   3. Dental teams.   4. Dental auxiliary
personnel.   I. Ryan, William J.   II. Title.
RK28.3.W54   617.6'01'07   81–19254
ISBN 0–8359–0897–6   AACR2
ISBN 0–8359–0896–8 pbk.

Editorial/production supervision and
      interior design by Norma M. Karlin
Manufacturing buyer: Ron Chapman

PRINTED IN THE UNITED STATES OF AMERICA

Dedicated to

Beverly and Mary Ryan,
C.B., and Yvonne Wiles,
and my best friends

CONTENTS

Foreword   xi

Preface   xv

Acknowledgments   xix

Introduction   1

PART I   PRINCIPLES OF HUMAN
            COMMUNICATION   11

Chapter 1   Types of Communication   13

            Intrapersonal Communication, 14
            Interpersonal Communication, 16
            Small-Group Communication, 22

Public Communication, 22
Intercultural Communication, 24
Mass Communication, 25
Summary, 26
Chapter Activities, 26
References, 27

Chapter 2   Theories and Models of Communication   28

Communication Models, 28
Factors Affecting Communication, 30
Communication Models for Dental
Auxiliaries, 32
Summary, 37
Chapter Activities, 37
References, 38
Bibliography, 38

PART II   PERSONAL ASPECTS OF
COMMUNICATION   41

Chapter 3   Perception   43

Perception of Self, 45
Perception of Others, 50
Personal Perception of Choices, 52
Summary, 60
Chapter Activities, 61
References, 62

Chapter 4   Role Behavior in the Dental Environment   63

Factors Influencing Roles, 64
Summary, 73
Chapter Activities, 74
References, 74

Chapter 5   Communication Choices   **76**

Personal Aspects of Communication, 77
Verbal Communication, 79
Vocal Communication, 84
Nonverbal–Nonvocal Communication, 89
Summary, 102
Chapter Activities, 103
References, 104
Bibliography, 105

**PART III   PROFESSIONAL ASPECTS OF
COMMUNICATION**   **109**

Chapter 6   First Impressions   **111**

Preparing for First Impressions, 113
Communication Review Questions, 120
Summary, 121
Chapter Activities, 121

**Chapter 7   Interviewing, Listening, and
Evaluating Responses**   **123**

Interviewing, 124
Two Typical Interviews, 130
Listening to the Patient, 133
Evaluating Patients' Responses, 136
Summary, 138
Chapter Activities, 139
Suggested References, 139

Chapter 8   Education, Motivation, and Persuasion   **141**

Learning Theories, 142
Two Learning Approaches, 147
Motivation, 148

Persuasion, 154
Learning/Motivating/Persuading:
A Practical Application, 157
Summary, 157
Chapter Activities, 160
References, 160
Bibliography, 161

PART IV   ORGANIZATIONAL COMMUNICATION
            AND THE DENTAL HEALTH TEAM   165

Chapter 9   Building a Good Dental Health Team   167

Factors Influencing Dental Health
Team Effectiveness, 169
The Needs of People on a
Dental Health Team, 172
Evolution of a Team, 173
Communication Networks, 176
Building a Successful
Dental Health Team, 179
The Dynamics of the
Dental Health Team, 183
Summary, 197
Chapter Activities, 198
References, 199

Chapter 10   Conflict Management and Problem Solving   200

Problem Solving, 201
Conflict, 206
Resolving Conflict, 212
Summary, 218
Chapter Activities, 219
References, 220
Bibliography, 220

Glossary   223

Index   227

FOREWORD

The state of the science of dentistry has reached the point at which it is now possible for almost everyone in an aware and motivated society to retain all their teeth for all their lives, in excellent condition in terms of comfort, function, health, and esthetics. Millions of dollars, dedicated to research in dentistry, have produced answers to the two essential reasons why people experience pain, suffering, disfigurement, and the loss of teeth: dental decay and/or periodontal disease. The other way these conditions are brought about is trauma—some form of accident. Research cannot prevent accidents, but it has provided the profession with a superb capability in restorative techniques and materials.

There is an obvious question: "If we have the capability to prevent virtually all the ravages of dental disease, why does it continue to plague us? Why don't we do something about it?" The answer is simply stated, but not simply achieved. It is to be found in the field of communication.

There are two particular areas in which communication must improve if the state of the art in dentistry (what is being delivered to the public) is to more nearly approach the state of the science (what is known and possible in the field). The first area concerns the education of the people in the profession. The dental schools are constantly attempting to improve their educational methods—their communication—so that the students go into practice with the highest possible ownership of what is known. The second category concerns educating and motivating the public so that people will be able to benefit from what is known about dentistry. It has been said that most people have money for what they realistically want; it is dentistry's challenge to help people want what they need.

Whether or not patients decide to have necessary dental treatment—or even assume the responsibility for their own dental health—depends not on the professional's ability or expertise in the delivery of high-quality care, but rather upon his or her skill in communicating the need for and importance of such care. Dentistry must come to occupy a significant position in people's priority schemes before its benefits can be realized. Sadly, most dental professionals have very little background, training, or orientation regarding communication of this need. Dentistry finds itself competing for the patient's time, attention, and money; the profession simply lacks expertise in advertising and in public education—what amounts to communication.

Training in technical dentistry is not enough; the dental professional also needs training in communication skills. Until this discrepancy is corrected, the public will not respond. This book, directed at the dental auxiliary, represents a long-needed step in the right direction; it will make a substantial inroad into solving the problem.

One of the most exciting approaches to solving the communication dilema focuses on the concept of teamwork in the private dental office. Many offices today are moving into a type of participative management in which every member of the dental team is actively involved in educating the public. But to be able to do this well, all the members—auxiliary personnel to the dentist—must sincerely believe in what they are attempting to communicate. This is the foundation of successful positive communication. Gimmicks are secondary; charts, models, pictures, and examples are merely tools, and are of little value if the person using them does not totally subscribe to their ultimate purpose—the delivery of the best dental care to people who know its value and want it. When such dedication to educate and serve is shared by all participants in an office community, this can lead to a meaningful synthesis of talents, training, and effort that is not possible to achieve through mechanical "book learning." In such an office community, beginning with this shared belief, the participants best combine their perceptions, skills, and temperaments to organize and present the advantages of dentistry to the public.

Communication is a multifaceted process. Two of the most important concerns in this process are the "messages" which the patient perceives consciously and those of which he or she is hardly aware, but receives subliminally or subconsciously. The auxiliary who is dedicated to providing optimum dental health care to patients will find this book invaluable in developing all aspects of communication techniques and approaches so that he or she can best transmit the message of the importance of dentistry to the recipient.

When the entire dental team shares this ability to communicate positively at every level, the patient benefits in terms of both dental health and attitude.

Within our profession today, there is an enormous capability to serve the dental health needs of the public. But the higher dimension of this capability consists of making the public aware of the need for and availability of this high-quality care. This can only be accomplished through better communication skills. The dentist today must surround him- or herself with a team whose members are able to focus their energy, time, thinking, and skills on positive communication as well as on technical procedures. Only then will patients know that they can indeed enjoy a lifetime of maximum dental health through a combination of their own efforts and the technical expertise of the dental team.

I applaud the authors, Cheryl B. Wiles and William Ryan, for adding this book to our professional armamentarium of knowledge, and I encourage all auxiliaries and dentists as well to read it and study it and own it.

Dr. LOREN MILLER, *Director*
The L. D. Pankey Institute for
Advanced Dental Education

PREFACE

As a dental auxiliary, you play an important role in helping others maintain their dental health. Dental professionals have come to realize that preventive dentistry requires more than technical clinical skills. In addition, the establishment of positive cooperative relationships with patients and with each other on the dental team is essential to providing optimum dental care. Communication is the key to developing and maintaining such relationships. This book is written for dental hygienists and dental assistants who have the interest and intent to better understand and practice effective communication in their personal and professional lives.

There are many popular books, scholarly research studies, and periodical articles written on the subject of communication. Very few deal with dentistry, and even fewer deal specifically with the work of dental assistants and dental hygienists. At the time of this writing, we are not aware of a single textbook on communication written specifically for dental auxiliaries. Yet, after scores of interviews with practicing dental assistants and dental hygienists, we have heard repeatedly that knowledge and ability in communication is crucial to the practice of preventive dentistry. This book is our invitation to all dental auxiliaries to learn and practice positive, productive, creative communication as individual persons and as dental professionals.

This book is unique because of a need for a textbook on communication specifically for dental auxiliaries written from a background of combined skills in dentistry and communication. While jointly working on a syllabus for a course in communication for dental hygienists, we looked in vain for such a textbook. Books available were either strictly general communication texts or were written primarily for dentists by dental professionals with a strong dental background but with little academic background in communication. While discussing this problem with a representative from Prentice-Hall, we found encouragement to turn our syllabus into the textbook which we felt would satisfy the need.

In working together on this book, we have combined the experience and academic background of two fields—dental hygiene and communication. Cheryl writes from her experience as a Registered Dental Hygienist and as an educator in a university dental school. Bill writes from his experience as a counselor in both church and medical settings and as an educator in the communication department of a liberal arts college. Neither has tried to become an "instant expert" in the other's field. Yet, each of us has learned a great deal from the other and has gained a new appreciation for the other's knowledge and experience. This is what we are passing along to you.

The contents of this book are divided into four parts. These include: Part I, "Principles of Human Communication"; Part II, "Personal Aspects of Communication"; Part III, "Professional Aspects of Communication"; and Part IV, "Organizational Communication and the Dental Health Team." We wanted to begin the subject of communication with some brief and basic theoretical information to make our readers conscious of some fundamental principles of communication that apply to experiences in daily living. The essence of being an effective communicator in preventive dentistry begins with oneself. Thus, Part II addresses the personal aspects of communication, including perceptions of self and others, roles, and verbal as well as nonverbal communication channels. With an understanding and awareness of oneself, the professional aspects of communication can be addressed. Part III concentrates on first impressions and their effect on patients, interviewing techniques, listening skills, and the roles of education, motivation, and persuasion. Finally, Part IV is concerned with the effectiveness of the dental health team, how to be a productive member, organizational communication, problem solving and conflict resolution.

Material selected for this book was chosen because of specific recommendations by persons active in the respective fields of communication and dentistry. It relates theory to realistic applications in dental offices and clinics. We have tried to balance intellectual and academic integrity with practical advice and real-life experiences of dental auxiliaries. Most of the examples in this book come from actual cases described for us by practicing dental assistants, dental hygienists, receptionists, dentists, and patients. For further reading in this field, we have included bibliographies at the end of each section.

Because both of the authors have been involved in continuing education, we have observed that it is often *after* receiving the basic dental education that dental auxiliaries discover the significance of communication skills. Thus, it can be used not only as part of a regular course curriculum but also as a reference book over the long-term practice of preventive dental care. It can stand alone as a text for a course in communication for dental auxiliaries or as a companion with other material in a general course in office practice management or human relations. And it could well be used as a resource for continuing education seminars. We think it has a wide variety of practical uses and believe that it is flexible enough for any learning situation and teaching style you might choose.

We believe that effective communication can be learned and that your knowledge of communication must be practiced daily in order for you to grow as a helping person. This book is a tool to help you in this growth. We hope that after using this book you will continue to evaluate your own communication behavior and continue to learn how to be an effective communicator in your personal relationships as well as in your professional life.

C.B.W

W.J.R.

ACKNOWLEDGMENTS

Many of our friends have offered their support and time to the preparation of this manuscript. We are indebted to the following Registered Dental Hygienists who shared with us their time, enthusiasm, and experiences: Lisa Telthorst, Nan Allen, Susan Stark, Mary Shelbey, and Rose Mary Minervini. The Certified Dental Assistants at the Universty of Missouri–Kansas City School of Dentistry were significant resources in the writing of this book. Our warm thanks and appreciation are extended to these women for their sincere interest. Many thanks are also appropriately given to the dental hygiene students, Class of 1981, University of Missouri–Kansas City School of Dentistry for their photographs—but particularly to the dental hygiene students from Teams 7 and 8 for their inspiration, support, and cooperation. Additional warm regards are extended to dentists Greg Seal, John Hughes, Eric Johnson, Ned Smith, Gary Zuck, and their professional staffs, as well as to Timi Martin and Lucille Heenan for their time and experiences. We wish to extend our appreciation to David Coats and Frank Hamilton for their photographic suggestions and professional services. We would personally like to acknowledge and thank our professional colleagues and friends, including Weslynn Martin, Chairperson, Department of Communication, Rockhurst College; Janice Woerth, Adele Eberhart, Mary Lu Andrews, Darryl Lefcoe, and Linda Platnik, dental hygiene educators. In addition, Sherry

Gound and Barbara Lambert, private dental hygiene practitioners, were valuable supporters in our endeavors. The interactions of all these individuals have been the most influential sources in the writing and organization of this manuscript. We thank Mary Ann Commick and Pamela McCandless for their typing and helpful suggestions.

COMMUNICATION FOR DENTAL AUXILIARIES

Introduction

Your thoughts and our thoughts about communication:

> I think communication is the most essential ingredient in making our team a success. Because we communicate quite well with one another we have established good professional and personal rapport, we understand where the other person is coming from when he or she reacts in a certain way, and most importantly, we trust each other. (*A practicing dental hygienist*)

> The one factor that keeps this dental corporation operating smoothly is communication. (*An office manager responsible for six dental practices*)

> Why am I successful as a dental assistant? Well, basically, it is because everyone in this office can openly communicate their desires, frustrations, etcetera." (*A practicing dental assistant*)

> Communication! That's the name of the game. We struggle with it all the time, but because we do it I really think we have an effective group of individuals delivering good dental care to our patients. (*A dentist in private practice*)

> There is only one thing that I can say that makes my work enjoyable and that is communication. When things go wrong around here, it all comes back to the fact that someone simply did not say what they needed or

1

how they could be helped. I don't know how to describe it, communication, but it is so important in all facets of my life. (*A dental receptionist in a private dental office*)

Communication, communication, communication . . . it is repeated over and over again by dental professionals as the essential factor in working on a team and being successful with patients. The importance of this art called communicating has been discussed in dental continuing education seminars by psychologists, dentists, human behavior researchers, psychiatrists, and educators in virtually all dental schools, dental society meetings, national professional meetings, local dental assisting and dental hygiene meetings across the country. They say to dental professionals:

Know thyself.

When patients feel love and trust among office staff, then they know you really care about them.

Help patients change their values by getting to know them.

If you listen to the conversations in the dental office, they are basically dialogues of the deaf. Listening is an interpersonal decision to be involved, not just with what someone is saying, but in terms of personal judgment, evaluation, or criticism.

Visualization is a powerful communication device.

Learn how to smile at your patients.

Listen to behavior, not just words. The real message is behavior.

Leadership is based on both skill and understanding in dealing with others.

One principle of human communication to remember is that the message sent is not always the message received.

Dental literature and health publications have a multitude of articles and books on the subject of communication. They appear in journal articles with titles like "Space: The Silent Language,"[1] "Talk Your Patient's Language,"[2] "Interpersonal Communication Skills Development: A Model for Dentistry,"[3] and "Touch: Comfort or Threat?",[4] to mention only a few. Titles such as *Communicate, On Caring, How Can We Reassure Patients?, People Reading, Communication and Persuasion, Interacting with Patients* are common resources in dental, dental hygiene, and dental assisting schools.

Why all this emphasis on communication? The answer is simple. People need other people to communicate. But why is communication important to you as a dental assistant or dental hygienist? Your professional responsibilities revolve around helping people receive dental care. First, you must learn to *communicate* with them. But you do not deliver dental care by yourself. You do not have all the skills necessary to render comprehensive treatment to patients. Thus, you *become a member of a team* that utilizes several resources to accomplish the task of delivering comprehensive dental care. For effective teamwork, *communication with team members* is inevitable as well as essential. Another truth about this art of communication is that when two or more individuals communicate with one another, perceptions, values, extent of comprehension, and ability to listen all have an important role in the success of the interaction. In all this discussion about the art of communication, the question "What is communication?" surfaces. Social scientists have tried to define communication but no universal definition exists because of its complexity. The definition varies according to the way it is to be used. Therefore, a place to begin is for you, as a dental auxiliary entering into the working world of dentistry, to create a definition of communication that is workable for *you*.

COMMUNICATION EXERCISE 1

Ask yourself, "What is communication?" and write your definition below:

Now consider the complexity of what you have just written. Communication has numerous sources and channels from which it is initiated, carried, and terminated. It has certain patterns and choices in various situations. They are available for us to use during every minute of the day. Reflect upon the conversation you have had with a classmate today. You transmitted some kind of message. How? By what means did you convey what you wanted the listener to receive? Was it a written or spoken message? Or was it perhaps a nonverbal one—such as a wink? How did the listener respond to you? Can you list some ways in which you sent messages to the other person?

1.

2.

3.

4.

What other factors in the conversation or the environment affected your communication with the listener (e.g., the smell of hot french fries, someone else talking, the noise of piped music)? List them.

1.

2.

3.

4.

The art of communicating involves innumerable factors. Indeed, the lists are almost endless when you begin to consider the environment that surrounds your communication processes. The dental environment, in itself, contributes specific noises, smells, sounds and objects that affect a dental auxiliary's communication channels and choices. Some are more influential than others, depending upon the specific dental treatment and the patient. The dental environment also affects the communication channels and choices you utilize during interactions with professional peers. The importance of communication for dental professionals that is stressed in continuing education seminars, journal articles, and books becomes more explicit when you begin to be open to what is occurring around you during daily communication with friends, teachers, and patients.

You were born into a world that bombards you with many noises, light sources, visual images, and a multitude of other physical stimuli. You spent most of your early infancy and childhood sorting out these stimuli and arranging them into some kind of logical order. Eventually you began to understand what they are all about and learned to respond in certain ways, influenced by the environment around you. All the giving and receiving you have initiated and responded to with family and friends has helped you to learn about who you are and what your identity is today. In turn, this identity you have chosen affects how you communicate. Ask yourself, "Who am I?"; Then complete the sentences below. They should be helpful as you begin to look at yourself and attempt to answer the question of who you are.

COMMUNICATION EXERCISE 2

My greatest strength is . . .
My greatest weakness is . . .
My greatest success is . . .
My greatest failure is . . .
I am most concerned with . . .
My greatest personal need is . . .
I am most aware of my . . .
People like me because . . .
I want to be . . .
Physically I appear to other people as . . .

Draw or describe a visual image of yourself

Communication scholars say that your self-image and value system have a great influence on how you communicate with other people. If you have a good feeling about yourself, then you will naturally choose positive channels of communication; if your self-image is not a positive one, your communication will reflect those feelings. This is of particular importance to remember when you hear mental health professionals say, "Know yourself," "Know your limitations," "Be kind to yourself," "Create bonding relationships in your life," "Don't be an emotional cripple." What you value also affects you in your professional role as a dental auxiliary and in your personal life as well.

COMMUNICATION EXERCISE 3

What four things do you value consistently in your life? Write them below:

1.

2.

3.

4.

Consider why you think the above four are important values in your life. Can you list reasons why you value them?

1.

2.

3.

4.

Now, reflect for a moment on your visits as a patient to a dental office. You undoubtedly had some kind of communication with the receptionist, dentist, dental assistant, and dental hygienist. Did you notice any particular characteristics about them as health professionals helping other people? Would they need to have any certain values about dental health to be successful in their job responsibilities? As we have already discussed, our values affect our communication with ourselves, our family, our friends, and patients. But how do these values influence your behavior?

COMMUNICATION EXERCISE 4

What behavioral characteristics do you practice that will be positive assets in your relationships with peers and patients in the dental office?

1.

2.

3.

4.

5.

6.

List four values you think are most important in your job responsibility as a dental auxiliary.

1.

2.

3.

4.

What factors have influenced you in incorporating these values into your professional role responsibility?

1 .

2.

3.

4.

5.

As you already may have experienced, conflicts often arise when two or more personalities and individuals become involved in communication in which a problem is not solved. Some dental journals have special columns dealing with communication problems in the dental office between staff members and patients. Dental continuing education courses have focused on interpersonal communication conflicts between dental health team members.

Have you considered specifically how you deal with communication problems that arise in your daily life or with patients? A colleague once said, "If I had a patient in the chair with whom I was not getting along very well, I tried to think of that person as a witch and that I had hidden her broom." Well, that is one answer, but not necessarily a very workable solution for every individual. Problem solving and conflict resolution are important skills requiring special communication techniques.

COMMUNICATION EXERCISE 5

How do you deal with conflicts that arise with your friends, family, or spouse? List them as specifically as you can:

1.

2.

3.

4.

5.

6.

What positive ways can you list to deal with problems involving your patients?

1.

2.

3.

4.

5.

6.

The communication choices and patterns that you choose to use are influential factors in your success with patients. Your ideas of what you think you should be doing for patients affects how you communicate with them and how they communicate with you in return. In essence, you influence the communication interactions around you. Learning to be influential takes a special consciousness on your part and special skills that can be learned. It is an ever-challenging process, as the following quotations exemplify:

> I am so frustrated at work that I am about ready to quit. It all started when the other dental hygienist, who is also the business manager, did not tell me that she was behind in her schedule and needed me to give her patient a fluoride treatment. It was a beautiful afternoon, I was done with my patients, so I just left. All she would have had to do was tell me she needed my assistance. Communication! It is so difficult! (*A dental hygienist*)

> I just don't agree with the dentist's philosophy. Our communication problem is a matter of values. (*A dental assistant*)

> Dental assistant is not talking to me. I wonder what problem we have . . . (*A dental receptionist in a dental office*)

> I just love my dentist. He is so concerned about my dental health. In fact, his entire staff really makes me feel welcome in the office, and I used to hate going to the dentist. I guess I have the same fears as everyone else . . . He always wants to know how I feel about his services. (*A patient*)

> I try not to let our communication channels get fouled up in this office. Getting along with one another in such a small space is bad enough without having some communication conflicts about who is supposed to do what and so on. (*A dentist in private practice*)

The remaining pages of this book are written to assist you in learning to be conscious of the communication skills that will make you a successful dental auxiliary. We will not tell you that you must believe that good communication is very important in your life. But we believe it, and this is why we attempt in the following chapters to bring to light some of the special skills and knowledge that will help you appreciate the importance of good communication in your professional and personal life. Before going on, look back at your definition of communication. With your own definition in mind, you are ready to read further, beginning with Part I on the Principles of Human Communication.

REFERENCES

1. Margaret L. Pluckhan, "Space: The Silent Language," *Nursing Forum*, VII, no. 4 (1968), 386–97.
2. Robert E. Gehrmann, "Talk Your Patients' Language," *Dental Management*, December 1979, 29–32.

3. J. Larry Hornsby, Lawrence J. Deneed, and David W. Heid, "Interpersonal Communication Skills Development: A Model for Dentistry," *Journal of Dental Education*, 39, no. 11 (1975), 728–32.

4. Lianne S. Mercer, "Touch: Comfort or Threat?" *Perspectives in Psychiatric Care*, 4, no. 6 (1966), 20–25.

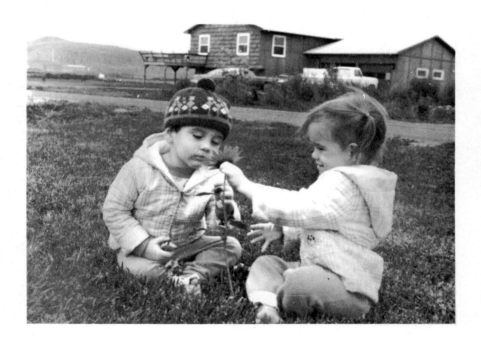

PRINCIPLES
OF HUMAN
COMMUNICATION

*Accurate and adequate communication
between groups and people will not in
itself bring about the millenium, but it is
a necessary condition for almost all forms
of social progress.*

Daniel Katz*

KEY POINTS

CHAPTER 1
Definition of Communication
Communication Situations
   intrapersonal
   interpersonal
   small-group
   public
   intercultural
Intrapersonal Communication
Aspects
   physiological process
   phychological process
Interpersonal Communication
   seven stages of dialogue

Small-Group Communication
Public Communication
Mass Communication

CHAPTER 2
Communication Models
Theoretical Models
   source-encoder-channel
   decoder-receiver-feedback
Factors Affecting Commun-
   ication
A Dental Auxiliary Model

Types of Communication

The practices of dental hygiene and dental assisting incorporate a vast array of professional skills, attitudes, values, goals, and philosophies. The breadth and depth of this array is sometimes overwhelming. To clarify the role of a dental auxiliary, let us focus our attention on the process of communication as it relates to these professions.

Definition of Communication

Communication can be defined as the process of sharing messages. This implies the ability to send and receive signals that are mutually understood. The middle part of the word communication, *-uni-*, denotes oneness—i.e., the bringing together of once-separate parts in order to have something in common.

Communication can be discussed in a variety of ways. For simplicity, we can begin by describing the situations in which it occurs. These include: (1) intrapersonal, (2) interpersonal, (3) small-group, (4) public, and (5) inter-cultural. The latter two situations may also include (6) mass communication, depending on the number of participants and the geographical distribution.

INTRAPERSONAL COMMUNICATION

Intrapersonal communication is the sending and receiving of messages within one person. This includes two general processes. One involves the activity within our central nervous system, which we shall call the physiological process. The other involves mental and intellectual activity, which we shall call the psychological process.

CENTRAL NERVOUS SYSTEM.   Three types of activity occur in the nervous system: sensory input, central connection and coordination, and motor output. We receive sensory input through sight, hearing, taste, touch, and smell. In the central nervous system these sensory impulses are not only received but are also associated within the brain and stored in our memory. Connections are made which may cause motor output, affecting muscular and glandular behavior. You might see an example of this process when a dental patient squints as the bright dental light shines into his eyes.

PSYCHOLOGICAL PROCESS.   The mental or psychological process occurs in the central connection and coordination activity and includes what we think about and how we symbolize. It is where meaning is developed and related to what we see, hear, and perceive happening in our world. Linguistic development occurs here, as we use words and grammar to formulate our thoughts, talk to ourselves, remember, and send messages to others. Semantic development helps us apply meaning to words and symbols. Human values, attitudes, role choices, beliefs, and goals are also developed in this process, eventually leading to decisions, and to action or inaction. When a dental auxiliary thinks of a person who seeks dental care as a "patient," a variety of meanings and role expectations develop as a result of the use of this particular word. "Patient" implies a person who is (a) not well, and (b) passive. Such assumptions and implications are drawn by intrapersonal communication.

The following example in Communication Exercise 1-1 illustrates a variety of intrapersonal communication activities. Of those we have just discussed, see how many you can recognize.

COMMUNICATION EXERCISE 1-1

A woman enters a dental office for a routine checkup. As she enters, she sees in the waiting room seashore pictures on pastel-colored walls, old magazines scattered on end tables, a few fidgety people seated in chairs around the room, a receptionist behind a glass window, and a sign that reads, "Please

Tell Receptionist You Are Here." She smells familiar odors which remind her of previous visits—not all pleasant, she recalls. After giving her name to the receptionist, she sits down. She wonders why there are never any interesting magazines to read. She would like to talk but everyone is silent, so she decides to remain silent. She begins to worry about whether or not she will have cavities. She crosses her legs and swings one foot back and forth, nervously; she picks up an old dental journal to get her mind off the pending examination.

What examples do you find that could be called *sensory input?*

What examples do you find that could be classified as *mental* or *psychological activity?*

What examples do you find that constitute *motor output?*

With the many stimuli, intrapersonal communication has resulted in a lot of physiological and psychological activity for the woman in this hypothetical illustration. How many could you identify?

Sensory input includes all the visual stimuli that bombard the woman as she enters the waiting room—pictures, furniture, wall colors, fidgety people, a sign, and the receptionist. Immediately, these stimulate her memory to formulate an image that is familiar and that begins to set an emotional mood for the pending dental exam. The odors reinforce this initial impression and further remind her of past experiences. She becomes very conscious of why she is here and begins to formulate decisions about how she will think and behave in this situation. The fidgety people seem to influence her to be likewise fidgety. She sets some rules for her own communication which, in turn, determine her motor output. She talks to the receptionist, sits down, decides to be silent (a nonverbal message in itself), and picks up a magazine to read. These are conscious, intrapersonal decisions, which will later have their consequences in how she meets and interacts with other members of the dental staff—dental hygienist, dental assistant, and dentist.

Dental auxiliaries who are aware of such intrapersonal communication in each of their patients are in a good position to relate to their patients with a positive sense of understanding and empathy.

INTERPERSONAL COMMUNICATION

Interpersonal communication usually refers to a situation wherein two people are sending and receiving messages together. It is also called "dyadic" communication. This is the context in which dental assistants and dental hygienists are likely to spend most of their professional time. Interpersonal communication is the most frequent form of communication used by professionals working together on a dental team as well as by professionals working with patients.

Understanding the complexity of *intra*personal communication is important in understanding the complexity of *inter*personal transactions. Consider this: two separate individuals with separate perceptions of themselves (their roles and their relationship to each other), bringing with them unique ethnic, social, linguistic, semantic, and educational backgrounds, living with different assumptions and values, face each other with a common goal that needs to be mutually understood and achieved. This is what happens each time you meet a patient in a dental environment. Multiply this situation by the approximate number of patients seen in a day (eight or more) and you can realize the importance of understanding some basic elements of effective interpersonal communication.

Interpersonal communication with patients, professional peers, and others in daily life is not a simple one-step process. Effective communication —getting across the message you *intend* to send and achieving the desired results—does not automatically occur just because you open your mouth and utter some words. If this is what you think communication includes you may frequently find yourself exclaiming, "But I explained it to her so clearly; why can't she understand it?" Effective communication involves several progressive steps. Clyde Reid has identified seven steps which lead to mutual action: (1) transmission, (2) contact, (3) feedback, (4) understanding, (5) acceptance, (6) internalization, and (7) action.[1]

Using Reid's steps you can follow interpersonal communication as it develops in our own diagram in Figure 1-1 to see how far you really have gone and where you have gotten bogged down. Following are our own explanations of this multiple step process, using Reid's terms as guides.

Transmission

Transmission is the sending of messages from one person to another. It is the use of any combination of the following means by which we send messages:

Verbal Communication	The use of words, in speaking or writing.
Vocal Communication	The use of sounds, such as the pitch and tone

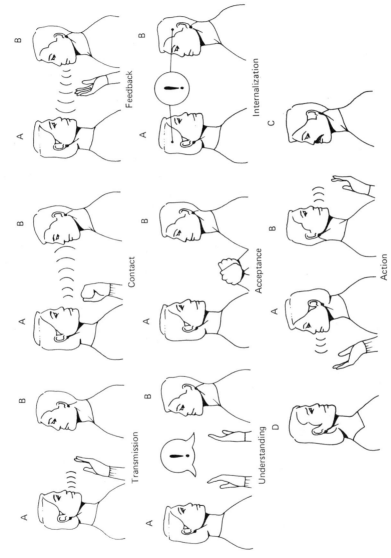

Figure 1-1. Seven steps of dialogue.

17

of voice, the volume of sound, and the articulation of sound into speech. A moan, a sigh, and a laugh are also vocal transmissions, any of which you could hear in a dental operatory.

Nonverbal–Nonvocal Communication

(1) The use of bodily movement and facial expressions (kinesics); (2) the placement of persons in relation to each other (proxemics), such as how close a dental auxiliary sits to a patient during an interview; (3) touch (tactile communication), such as the firmness or gentleness of your hands on a patient's jaw and mouth; and (4) the use of the sense of smell, such as the use of mouthwash, or the aroma of disinfectant used to clean the sink and suction. Keeping in mind that vocal communication may be either verbal or nonverbal, dental auxiliaries need to be aware of the variety of ways messages are transmitted, both by themselves and by others.

Contact

Contact is the sensory reception of your transmission, physiologically, by the other person. The person hears, sees, smells, feels, or tastes. Unless there are physical handicaps, all of these senses are active; the latter three are probably more active for a patient during dental treatment than during other times of his or her daily activities. But contact does not mean understanding! For example, hearing is not the same as listening. You can hear a person speaking but not comprehend the meaning (semantics) of the words. If you tell a patient that he has gingivitis he may *hear* the sound of the word and *see* that you are talking to him. This is contact. But if he has never heard the word "gingivitis" it is likely that he will have no idea what it is that you are describing. He may infer from your facial expression and the tone of your voice that something is undesirable in his oral cavity. But that is about as close to understanding the meaning of that dental terminology as he can get. You, as the one who transmitted the message, will need to rely on the next step to determine in what way this inital contact has been perceived.

Feedback

Feedback is the response or message returned to the original sender of the message. It lets person A know what person B has heard and how person B understands the initial transmission. If, for example, you tell a patient that he needs to have a cavity filled he may send a strong nonverbal message back by clinching his fist so hard that his knuckles turn white. Or, it can be a simple verbal exchange such as "It looks like you have been flossing regularly," followed by "Yes." Feedback allows the originator of a message to adjust the communication so that subsequent transmissions will be more effective. It is simply "knowledge of results."[2] In interviewing, it is essential for the health professional to pay close attention to feedback from the patient in order to fully understand his or her needs. In learning, attending to feedback from a teacher allows a student to know how to make necessary adjustments for improvement.

Understanding

Understanding means that the person to whom a message has been transmitted comprehends the language (linguistics) and meaning (semantics) of what is said. The language may be ethnic slang or it may be technical, professional dental terminology. Either way, is it mutually understood? Recall our example in the contact step, in which we suggested that if you tell a patient he has gingivitis when he may not know the meaning of the word, you will need to ask the patient if he understands what that is. If he says, "I'm not sure; I think so," you would need to explain this in terms he can understand. For example, you might say, "Gingivitis is an inflammation of the gums. Do you notice any soreness here? Is it tender when I touch it?" Through facial expressions, a few words, or the nodding of his head he may acknowledge that he now understands more clearly what you mean. Keep in mind that both spoken and unspoken messages are sent and received, and it is important that both you and the patient understand both the verbal and nonverbal messages of each other. He may wonder why you frown when you use the word "gingivitis." Does this mean that he has a very serious disease which will require painful or expensive preventive dental care? Understanding both spoken and unspoken messages is important. When both persons do acknowledge a mutual understanding of what each has transmitted, you may move to the next step.

Acceptance

Acceptance means that the initial message is seen as valid—not necessarily valid for person B but valid for person A who sent the message. A patient might say, "Yes, I agree that using dental floss each day is a good idea." Saying this is not agreeing to use dental floss; it is acceptance of the validity of this concept.

Internalization

Internalization occurs when the thoughts and messages of person A become a part of the thoughts and messages of person B in an interpersonal transaction. A *common* idea, goal, perception, or concept is held by each. Each "owns" the idea as it becomes a part of his or her own thinking and acting behavior. An example of this would be if the patient whom you just persuaded to accept the idea of using dental floss in regular daily dental care goes home and honestly attempts to persuade others that this is a good practice.

Action

Action is the final step in interpersonal communication. Each person agrees to take—and does take—common action. A patient, for example, having discussed the value of using dental floss, now actually will begin to use it regularly. It could be argued that communication is not actually complete until some observable action occurs which corresponds with the initial transmission of a message.

These seven steps in interpersonal communication can best be called *dialogue* because they involve both parties and include consensus arrived at through mutual interaction.

In the following illustration in Communication Exercise 1-2, can you identify each of the seven stages of dialogue? If you correctly label the seven stages as they are itemized in the exercise, you will realize that in dialogue it takes time to accomplish a consensus. It takes a while to reach acceptance and internalization of an idea. Simply telling patients what's wrong with them with your own terminology will not necessarily result in their understanding it or doing anything about it. Dialogue helps achieve consensus.

COMMUNICATION EXERCISE 1-2

In the left-hand column are numbers denoting each of the seven stages of dialogue, as it occurs in the case described in the right-hand column. Test your memory concerning each of these stages by reading the conversation and then identifying the stage by its label. If you cannot recall what a stage is called, refer back to the previous explanation of dialogue in this chapter.

STAGE OF DIALOGUE		CONVERSATION
I	DENTAL AUXILIARY:	Bill, as I probe I find 4-mm and 5-mm pockets around the distals of your mandibular posterior teeth.
II III	PATIENT:	(Silence. He wrinkles his brow, indicating that he heard the statement yet implying that he is not sure what it means.)
I	AUXILIARY:	What this means is that your gums around the backs of your bottom teeth are bleeding spontaneously.

I, II, III, & IV	PATIENT:	Do you mean that I have some kind of disease?
I, II, III, & IV	AUXILIARY:	Yes, that's right.
	PATIENT:	Is it serious?
	AUXILIARY:	Yes, it is serious; but there are several things we can do. (Explanation follows.)
V	PATIENT:	What I hear you saying is that I need to religiously use dental floss, toothbrush, and perio aid every day. And I will see you again in two weeks for what you call "preventive plaque score exam"?
V	AUXILIARY:	Yes, that's right. Do you think that's something you can do?
VI	PATIENT:	Oh, sure. Yeh, I really want to get my mouth back in shape. I'd better do it, hadn't I?
	AUXILIARY:	(Smiles.)
VII	PATIENT:	(Leaves, and over the next two weeks, does what he agreed to do.)

Assertiveness and Authoritativeness

Interpersonal communication may take place "colored," as it were, by one of two common attitudes which cause the communication to be less of a dialogue and more of a monologue. These attitudes are assertiveness and authoritativeness. *Assertive* behavior occurs when one person confronts another, very honestly and directly, and without fear of what the other might feel or expect of that person in return. Although not aggressive, assertiveness is generally a monologue. Dr. Sharon Helm, who teaches assertiveness training, describes this form of communication as standing up for one's legitimate rights without infringing on the rights of others—for example, the right to say no, the right to ask for what you want, and the right to make mistakes. You may need to tell a patient that he has traumatic occlusion causing localized areas of periodontitis, even if he does not want to hear about his condition. *Authoritarian* communication is also a monologue, occurring, for example, when a person perceives herself as having more power or expertise than another, and consequently makes demands, issues orders, or makes assumptions about the expectations of the other. In this situation, decisions are unilateral, not mutual. Authoritarian communication may be necessary in times of emergency and when decisions need to be made quickly and concretely. A dentist may need to give instructions to an auxiliary in order to accomplish a particular dental procedure without the need for dialogue. Likewise, a dental hygienist may need to give authoritative instructions to a patient as a means of persuasion. Under such conditions, authoritarian communication may be an acceptable choice. However, authoritarian behavior is not always received in a positive way, especially if it is the preferred style of a dental professional on a regular,

daily basis. Sometimes dentists are accused by auxiliaries of being authoritarian. Dentists, in turn, sometimes call dental hygienists "prima donnas"
when they are communicating in an authoritarian manner. If you were the
one to tell a patient that he needed a full set of radiographs, which form of
interpersonal communication would you use—dialogue, assertiveness, or
authoritativeness?

More will be said about interpersonal communication in subsequent
chapters.

SMALL–GROUP COMMUNICATION

Communication in small groups (three to about seventeen persons) can occur
for different reasons, including information sharing, decision making, problem solving, therapy, and social entertainment. Staff meetings in clinics,
hospitals, and dental offices most often involve the first three reasons. For
whatever reason a group meets, each group has its own peculiar set of
behavioral patterns. These *group dynamics* can be observed and managed.
Factors affecting the dynamics include the roles of people in the group, the setting, the amount of time available, the goal or task of the personal moods and
feelings of each individual, the rules for getting the task done, and even the
way in which people are physically positioned in relation to one another in the
group. More will be said about group interaction in Part IV.

PUBLIC COMMUNICATION

Speeches given to audiences and lectures given in educational settings are two
examples of public communication. Dental assistants and dental hygienists
would most likely find themselves involved in planning and preparing a
speech for such occasions as a panel presentation to a community organization or on radio or television; giving a talk with visual aids and demonstra-
tions in educational settings, from preschool through graduate professional
school; or presenting a paper or demonstration at a continuing education con-
ference for dental auxiliaries. Basically, a public speech is given for one of
three purposes: to entertain, to inform or educate, or to persuade or motivate.
A speaker integrates the five following skills in presenting information in a
public communication:

1. *Organization* of main ideas into an easily followed pattern.
2. *Development of style* in the use of words to convey the ideas in ways
   that can be understood by the particular audience.

3. *Development of content*, including data, statistics, examples, case studies, and quotes from authorities and current sources to give substance to the speech and to support the main points.
4. *Use of logic* and the avoidance of fallacies such as half-truths, stereotypes, using false causes to explain problems, and so forth.
5. *Delivery* of the speech using a pleasing tone and speaking loud enough for all to hear (or directed into the microphone rather than away from it), articulating speech sounds clearly, speaking at a rate that is easy to follow, and using vocal inflections that express appropriate moods and emotions for the topic.

A speech usually is prepared in advance, either in a full manuscript form that has been practiced several times so it will not need to be read directly from the pages, or in an outline form on note cards or a single sheet of paper to keep the speaker on the track and to make sure important material is quoted correctly.

Such public communication may not be a frequent activity for a dental auxiliary early in the profession. However, as you join professional dental societies and become active in community affairs, public speaking will become at least an infrequent form of communication, and it will require some preparation and skill. Also, simply knowing the five elements listed above will help you listen more carefully to lecturers and speakers. Most good speeches have three basic, main sections:

I. Introduction

II. Body of the speech

III. Conclusion

Some speech teachers summarize this by telling students that this means to "Tell 'em what you're going to tell 'em. Tell 'em. Then, tell 'em what you've told 'em." Whether you are a speaker or a listener, knowing that a speech should be organized in an easily followed pattern will assist the total communication process of sending and receiving the message with understanding.

It also helps to be able to identify very early in the speech what the purpose of the speaker is (to entertain, to inform, or to persuade) and what is the main proposition that will guide the rest of the speech—that is, what is it the speaker expects the listeners to think, learn, be able to do or change as a result of the speech. Whether you are speaker or listener, knowing this early in the speech is important. Speakers who do not do this frequently have audiences that are not sure what it is they have heard when it is all over. Listeners who cannot identify the main proposition sometimes get fooled into doing things they later regret, simply because they did not listen carefully or analytically to the speaker, or the speaker did not make use of the five skills listed above to present their information.

FAVORABLE TOWARD	THE SPEAKER	THE TOPIC	THE OCCASION
Indifferent about	''	''	''
Simply curious about	''	''	''
Hostile toward	''	''	''

Figure 1–2. Audience attitudes.

Keep in mind, too, that one major difference between interpersonal communication and public communication is that usually a public speech or lecture is a monologue, in which one person speaks to many. For the speaker, the complexities of interpersonal communication are multiplied by the number of listeners in the audience. This makes the communication process more difficult because feedback from each person may indicate a slightly different understanding of what the speaker is saying. Trying to adjust to each person's feedback in a large crowd is almost impossible in the same way it can be done in interpersonal dialogue. However, speakers who understand their audiences usually can deliver messages that are commonly understood, accepted, and internalized.

In order to adapt to an audience, a speaker can try to get a general idea about how the audience feels. The chart in Figure 1-2 illustrates various attitudes which an audience might have in a public communication situation.

This information helps the speaker to determine how to establish some common ground toward the audience. If, for example, an audience is hostile toward a speaker, the speaker can deal not so much on his or her own credibility but deal directly in a logical way with the topic, thus drawing audience attention away from the speaker and toward something they all have in common, the topic.

All these elements are fundamental to public communication. This textbook does not deal with public communication beyond this chapter. However, many of the elements of education and persuasion discussed in Chapter 8 apply to interpersonal communication as well as to public communication. Dental auxiliaries who become active in leadership roles in their local, state, and national dental associations and professional societies soon realize the importance of developing skills in public speaking.

INTERCULTURAL COMMUNICATION

Intercultural communication is communication between people who have different cultural backgrounds. These differences may occur in the areas of language; race; ethnic origin and expression; religion; ceremonies; form of government; traditions and customs; types of seasonal sports; work and leisure expectations; use of time, food, economics, and dress; and so forth. In spite of the potential for world travel and communication, humankind is not one uniform family living in one common village. To acknowledge and respect cultural differences is a necessary preliminary to intercultural communication.[3]

In dental practice, the possibility for intercultural interaction is great. It occurs not only in dental-school clinics serving metropolitan communities but also on military bases and in any instance in which a professional may move from one locale to another. For example, a black dentist from New Jersey may establish a private practice in a rural all-white community in Nebraska where no local dentist has practiced before. Language, dental-care habits, dress, use of time, racial stereotypes, and professional ethics may all contribute to special challenges and adaptations that could involve intercultural communication behavior.

MASS COMMUNICATION

Interrelated with both public and cultural aspects of communication is mass communication. As a dental auxiliary you may have opportunities to appear on television or speak on radio, participate in making movies for general education, record messages on audiotape or videotape, or write books and journal articles. Mass communication allows messages to be shared over a large geographical area, and to be repeated over a long period of time. One disadvantage of communication using electronic, photographic, and print media is that there is little chance for dialogue. It is basically a one-way communication, with little immediate feedback. Although some cable television systems do allow immediate feedback, most forms of mass communication are limited to monologue. There are many advantages, however. The use of mass media to inform, educate, and persuade has great creative potential for any special-interest group wishing to communicate to a large and/or distant audience. Debating the public issue of fluoridated water on a radio talk show is a case in point. Another use is closed-circuit instructional television (ITV) used in clinical education and observation. University and community college dental libraries can store videotapes of clinical practice procedures and surgical techniques for multiple and individual use.

Currently, all commercially licensed television and radio stations are required by the Federal Communications Commission to provide free public service time for not-for-profit organizations. Preventive dental care and related topics could be discussed through public service announcements (PSAs) taped for broadcast on radio or television. Dental hygiene and dental assistant associations can take advantage of this use of mass communication in creative ways.

Having discussed the various types of communication, we are now ready to move on to theories and models which will help to describe and illustrate how communication occurs.

SUMMARY

Communication is the process of sharing messages. It implies the ability to send and receive signals that are mutually understood. There are six important communication situations: intrapersonal, interpersonal, small-group, public, intercultural, and mass communication. Intrapersonal communication is the sending and receiving of messages within one person. It involves a physiological and psychological process. Interpersonal communication (also called dyadic communication) refers to a situation wherein two people are sending and receiving messages together. Effective interpersonal communication involves seven steps as outlined by Clyde Reid: (1) transmission, (2) contact, (3) feedback, (4) understanding, (5) acceptance, (6) internalization, and (7) action. The completion of these seven steps is called *dialogue.* Transmission is the sending of messages from one person to another. It involves vocal, verbal and nonverbal-nonvocal communication choices. Contact is the sensory reception of the transmission, physiologically, by the other person. Feedback is the response or message returned to the original sender of the message. Understanding means that the person to whom a message has been transmitted comprehends the language and meaning of what has been said. Acceptance means that the initial message is seen as valid from the person who sent it. Internalization occurs when the thoughts and messages of the sender become a part of the thoughts and messages of the person receiving the message. Action occurs when each person agrees to take common action in relation to the message sent and received. Other types of interpersonal communication include assertive and authoritarian communication. Small-group communication, intercultural communication, and mass communication also influence the communication choices of dental assistants and dental hygienists within the context of the dental environment.

CHAPTER ACTIVITIES

1. Name each type of communication discussed in this chapter and give for each one an example involving a dental auxiliary.
2. Using a personal situation involving you and another person, evaluate an interpersonal encounter by (a) listing each of the seven steps of interpersonal communication, then (b) describing your actual communication behavior for each step. (If you did not reach certain steps, list them but leave the description space blank.)

3. From your own experience as a dental patient, list as many nonverbal forms of communication as you can remember, being as specific as possible (i.e., "I gripped the armrest when I heard the sound of the drill").

REFERENCES

* Daniel Katz, "Psychological Barriers to Communications," *The Annals of the Academy of Political and Social Science*, 250 (March 1947), 17. Used with permission.

1. Clyde Reid, *The Empty Pulpit* (New York: Harper & Row, 1967), pp. 68–72; see also Melvin L. DeFleur and Otto N. Larsen, *The Flow of Information: An Experiment in Mass Communication* (New York: Harper & Row, 1958), pp. 4–6 and chap. 10, "Compliance as a Test of Effective Communication"; and Larry A. Samovar and Edward D. Rintye, "Interpersonal Communication: Some Working Principles," in *Small Group Communication: A Reader*, ed. Robert S. Cathcart and Larry A. Samovar (Dubuque, Ia.: W. C. Brown, 1970), pp. 278–88.

2. John Annett, *Feedback and Human Behavior* (Baltimore: Penguin Books, 1969), p. 60.

3. See L. S. Harms, *Intercultural Communication* (New York: Harper & Row, 1973), pp. 34–43; and Edward T. Hall, *The Silent Language* (New York: Doubleday, 1959).

Theories and Models of Communication

2

We have looked at six communication situations and their related forms and components. What can be said about communication that might apply to *all* of these situations? Is there one way of understanding the human communication process which could help a dental hygienist or dental assistant understand each daily situation clearly?

COMMUNICATION MODELS

An easy way to begin to answer these questions is look at some basic "models" of how the human communication process works. Understanding such models can help dental auxiliaries deal with daily communication transactions as they occur and as they are discussed in the remainder of this book.

Wilbur Schramm's Models

Three models developed by Wilbur Schramm are among many developed by communication theorists to explain the process of human communication.[1] In Figure 2-1 Schramm's communication model includes these basic components: source, encoder, signal, decoder, and destination.[2]

The *source* is where the message begins. The message begins in the brain and is transmitted by speech, body movements, writing, art, music, and other audible and/or visible means. Because the sender of the message intends for

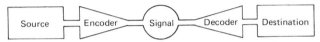

Figure 2–1. Wilbur Schramm communication model.

another person to understand it, the message is put into an intelligible "code," such as language—i.e., "it is encoded." At that point it becomes a message signal being sent through some medium or media, such as sound waves or light waves. Sometimes this is referred to as the "channel" through which the message flows. Then the message or "code" is decoded. That is, the language is heard and interpreted, once it is received. Once it is interpreted, it has arrived at its destination.

In order for the source to know how much of the message has been understood, the person who is the "destination" of the initial message acknowledges in some way what has been received. This, as has been discussed under interpersonal communication in Chapter 1, is "feedback," or knowledge of results. This allows adjustment in the communication so that subsequent messages will be better understood. Figure 2–2, Schramm's feedback model, shows this process by means of arrows going in circular directions, indication that each person has an encoding and decoding task.[3]

All this happens within the "field of experience" of each person (Figure 2–3). Some parts of the person's field of experience may overlap. The word "communication" itself implies sharing something in common, thus the overlapping ellipses in Schramm's model in Figure 2–3.[4]

Understanding the parts of these models may help us understand how communication works and why it does not always result in what we assume will happen. Messages can be "filtered" at many stages in the process. However, as Watzlawick, Beavin, and Jackson have shown, "*One cannot* not *communicate.*"[5] Whenever two or more people are together, communication occurs in some form.

To illustrate how this model fits a daily conversation in a dental office, a dental hygienist may say to a dentist, "Mrs. Jones has periodontitis. The

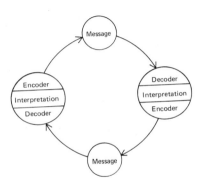

Figure 2–2. Wilbur Schramm feedback model.

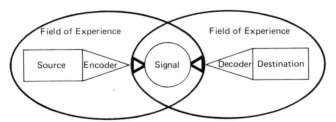

Figure 2–3. Wilbur Schramm field of experience model.

X-rays show significant interproximal bone loss. I get readings of 5 to 7mm generally throughout the posteriors on both the maxillary and mandibular arches. I really don't think she can adequately clean the areas with flossing and brushing."

The dental hygienist who says this has first made some decisions. She has chosen the language to use that will convey her thoughts as accurately as possible to another person whom she assumes will understand the words she uses. She makes this decision based on her own education and experience. Then her brain causes her vocal tract to speak the words and sentences she has chosen. Thus, the source, the hygienist, has encoded her message. As she speaks, the air in the room allows the sound to reach the ears of the dentist, who then instantly selects the sounds which he recognizes and the words he knows and the ideas he understands. This reception and selection process is the decoding process; it allows the hygienist's ideas to reach the destination. When the dentist has acknowledged what he has understood, the hygienist can either change the original message for clarity or simply go on to a new point. The dentist's acknowledgement is feedback. The two persons eventually come to some understanding of each other within their own fields of dental experience, which provides them at some point with *common ground.* They may have different backgrounds, but within some of their experience they have a few things in common which assist them in their communication.

FACTORS AFFECTING COMMUNICATION

David Berlo says that the fidelity of a message is affected by at least four factors: (1) communication skills, (2) attitudes, (3) knowledge level, and (4) position within a sociocultural system.[6] Because each person develops these to different degrees and under different circumstances, effective communication becomes quite a complex art. Communication skills include all the ways in which people send messages to others. It is a false assumption that because people have been to school, held jobs, and associated with others from infancy through adulthood they have developed high competency in communication abilities. For some, casual conversation comes easily; for others it is a difficult accomplishment. Some know how others perceive them and others seem to be oblivious of this. Attitudes also influence the ability to communicate well. An indifferent attitude on the part of one person can easily weaken the interest which a listener has in what the speaker has to say. An open and supportive attitude by one toward the other may cause the receiver of a message to listen carefully and openly. How much each person knows about the subject he or she is discussing, as in the case of a dental auxiliary talking with a dentist, will affect the fidelity of their communication, just as it will when a dental professional talks to a patient who has little understanding of dental procedures. And the way people see each other in terms of social relationships will also affect the communication. Dental professionals and others in medical fields often perceive themselves as "higher" in social status than those who are in semiskilled work. If such a feeling is present in an interpersonal encounter, it will influence the way in which each one "sees" the other and affect the choices of words, eye contact, and other means of communicating. Your understanding of a basic theoretical model of the communication process will help you analyze each encounter more clearly. We agree with Eleanor Hein, educator and nurse, that in the health professions the *knowledge* of the communication process itself affects communication behavior.[7]

COMMUNICATION EXERCISE 2-1

From your own experience and knowledge, list the information that fits each of the elements of Schramm's communication models (Figures 2-1, 2-2, and 2-3), itemized below.

SOURCE. (List as many aspects of your own identity as you can which influence your communication. Include education, beliefs, sociocultural background, attitudes, and language styles.)

ENCODING. (List all the ways, verbally and nonverbally, in which you tell others about yourself and your goals in life.)

CHANNEL. (Name all the various media which you use to send messages—e.g., speech, memos, telephone, etc.)

(continued)

COMMUNICATION EXERCISE 2-1 (Contd)

DECODING.   (Name the things others do to help you understand what they are trying to convey to you. Use your own words to describe this.)

FEEDBACK.   (List as many ways you can think of which you use to let other persons know how you understand their messages sent to you.)

COMMUNICATION MODELS FOR DENTAL AUXILIARIES

Chapter 1 introduced six types of communication, with descriptions of each as they relate to dental practice. Thus far in this chapter, some theoretical models of communication have been introduced. [8] Models help to illustrate the process of human communication and should be applicable to any human encounter. A model designed specifically for dental-health-care delivery might make the models discussed in this chapter even more applicable for use with patients. The model shown in Figure 2-4 gives substance to Schramm's models as they apply to the work of a dental auxiliary. Each part of this model corresponds to each element in Schramm's models in Figures 2-1, 2-2, and 2-3. You can use such a model to understand daily professional interactions with patients. This model is limited to professional-patient communication. Communication between dental professionals working as a team will be discussed in the last part of this book.

Five E's, Five S's, an R, and a P

Another way of understanding the model for dental auxiliaries is shown in the pictorial model in Figure 2-5. Here, both the dental auxiliary and the patient are viewed as sources encoding messages as well as receivers decoding messages. Each sends feedback to the other. Both are affected by their mutual fields of influence. To help make this model easier to remember, we use terms which you might find easy to remember in this way:

5 E's, 5 S's, an R, and a P.

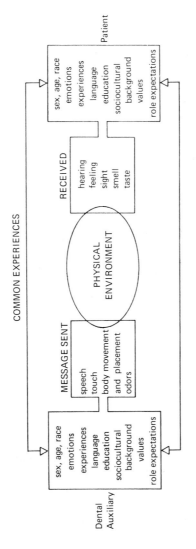

Figure 2-4. Dental auxiliary communication model.

33

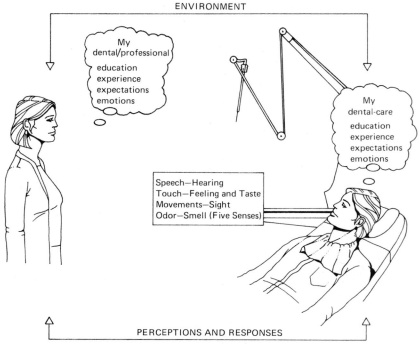

ENVIRONMENT

My dental/professional
education
experience
expectations
emotions

My dental-care
education
experience
expectations
emotions

Speech—Hearing
Touch—Feeling and Taste
Movements—Sight
Odor—Smell (Five Senses)

PERCEPTIONS AND RESPONSES

Figure 2–5. Dental auxiliary pictorial model.

Each person in this model bases his or her communication behavior on the following five E's:

Education   Dental education for hygienists and assistants in dental schools, community colleges, and vocational schools; dental health instruction for the patient in elementary schools and from dental professionals during appointments throughout life.

Experience   Actual practice in clinics and offices, variety of behaviors are observed by professionals; patient experiences, both positive and negative, create expectations.

Expectations   Professionals have professional standards and expectations of themselves and of their patients; patients have expectations of the dental hygienist and dental assistant, based on past experiences (personal concern is an example).

Emotions   Professionals have feelings brought on by the events of the day, feelings about individual patients and about themselves;

patients have emotions such as fear, anxiety, hope, and helplessness.

Environment The physical environment includes the room lighting, colors on the walls, background music, dental equipment and instruments, odors related to dental operatories, the comfort of the chair, and decorations on the walls.

These "five E's" help determine how messages are sent and received. Messages are received by the "five S's," the five senses, which have their corresponding physiological message-sending encoders.

FIVE SENSES CORRESPONDING ENCODER & EXAMPLE

Sight *Body movements* (kinesics), and *body placement* (proxemics), as well as the *use and placement of various physical objects*, such as dental instruments, in view of the patient.

Hearing *Speech*, including both verbal and vocal aspects.

Feeling *Touch* (tactile communication), such as handling mouth and jaw.

Taste *Placement of substances in the oral cavity*, such as fluoride and polishing paste.

Smell *Odors* emitted from body and mouth, chemicals used in the dental environment. Perfume, deodorant, mouthwash, and the smell of freshly washed hands are examples which patients may notice.

The five E's and the five S's (senses) combine to determine the P and the R, the *perceptions* and the *responses* of each person. Perceptions and responses, in turn, affect the communication behavior of both persons. *Perceptions* correspond to the encoding process in Schramm's models. Perception is the way we interpret the messages which one or more of the five senses have received. When we hear someone speaking, the sense of hearing alone does not tell us what the sounds mean. It is the way our brain processes this information, applying it to our own knowledge experience and emotions, which give us a picture of what has been heard. In turn, we respond to what we have heard and perceived. In the Schramm models, this corresponds to feedback. It is the way we let the other person know what we heard and perceived. These perceptions and responses keep the communication process going, making it a dynamic, rather than static, form of human behavior.

Depending on the circumstances, each of these elements has some degree of influence on the effectiveness of communication to the delivery of preventive dentistry. As a dental auxiliary, you must be alert to the uniqueness of each communication situation and understand, as clearly as possible, how all these variables influence the effectiveness of your transactions and your procedures. Being aware of the aforementioned five E's, five S's, the P and the R can help you analyze each situation for its unique characteristics. Once you understand the situation, the easier it will be for you to decide what steps to take for the effective communication that will help create a successful transaction with patients and other members of the dental health team.

In the following hypothetical situation you can follow the communication process by applying the Communication Model for Dental Auxiliaries to the various elements in the situation.

5 E's, 5 S's, P, & R	DIALOGUE
The Auxiliary's *EDUCATION* and *EXPERIENCE* influence her initial contact and message with the patient. Patient *RESPONDS* to the CDA's smile and tone of voice received by *SIGHT* and *HEARING* and forms a *PERCEP-TION* of the CDA which allows him or her to talk freely. Patient's *EMOTIONS* are based both on the CDA's *EXPERIENCE* and on her present *EXPECTATIONS*. Auxiliary controls the *ENVI-RONMENT* for the patient's comfort, helping her to *PER-CEIVE* an orderly and comfortable *ENVIRONMENT* through the *SENSES* of *SIGHT*, *HEAR-ING*, and *FEELING*.	A Certified Dental Assistant with an Associate of Arts degree in dental assisting from a metropolitan community college greets a patient in the doorway of a dental office. "Hello, Mrs. S_____. You may come in now. Please go to the room at the end of the hall, on your left." Mrs. S_____ smiles and says, "Oh, yes; the same one I was in last time when I had my wisdom tooth removed. Remember?" The CDA replies, "Have you had any complications from the extraction?" "No," says the patient, "I'm just here for a checkup and I don't know of any problems this time, thank goodness!" The CDA smiles and walks with Mrs. S_____ into the operatory, helps to adjust the dental chair to a comfortable position for the patient, and affixes the napkin carefully and gently around patient. She arranges the dental instruments carefully and neatly on the tray in front of the patient and asks if she is comfortable. Mrs. S_____ smiles and says, "Yes, thank you—you always make me feel relaxed when I'm here."

Now that you are aware of a few ways in which the communication process can be described in theory and illustrated in models, you are ready to apply these theories and models to specific communication situations.

SUMMARY

In this chapter, you have been introduced to three communication models by Wilbur Schramm. The basic components include source, encoder, signal, decoder, and destination. The source is where the message begins. The message is then put into an intelligible code such as language. The person sending the messages is called the encoder. Once it is encoded, the message is sent through some kind of medium such as sound waves. Then the message is decoded. The person receiving the message is the decoder. Once the message is interpreted, it has arrived at its destination. In order for the source to know how the message has been understood, the person who is the destination acknowledges in some way what has been received (feedback). All these basic components occur within a field of experience of each person receiving as well as sending the messages. Social scientists have shown that *"one cannot not communicate."* This means that whenever two or more people are together, communication occurs in some form. The fidelity of a message, according to David Berlo, is affected by at least four factors: communication skills, attitudes, knowledge level, and position within a sociocultural system. Each of us develops these factors to different degrees and under different circumstances. In the communication model for dental auxiliaries, the dental auxiliary and the patient are viewed as sources encoding messages as well as receivers decoding messages. Each sends feedback to the other and both are affected by mutual fields of experience. To understand the model, it is easier to remember that each person in this model bases his or her communication behavior on the following: education, experience, expectations, emotions, and environment. These help determine how messages are sent and received. Most of us receive messages by using the five senses: sight, hearing, feeling, taste, and smell. A combination of any or all help create effective communication abilities within all of us.

CHAPTER ACTIVITIES

1. Draw one of Schramm's communication models and label each part. Illustrate it further with a real experience you have had to deal with in communicating with fellow classmates.
2. Based on your understanding of the models, either discuss with another person or write a paragraph explaining why *"One cannot not communicate."*
3. List the "five E's" and give an example based on your own personal experiences in the dental office as a patient. Consider your responses to and perceptions of each.

REFERENCES

1. Wilbur Schramm, "How Communication Works," in *The Process and Effects of Mass Communication,* ed. Wilbur Schramm (Urbana, Ill.: University of Illinois Press, 1955), pp. 4–8.
2. Ibid., p. 6.
3. Ibid., p. 8.
4. Ibid., p. 8.
5. Paul Watzlawick, Janet Helmick Beavin, and Don D. Jackson, *Pragmatics of Human Communication* (New York: W. W. Norton & Co., Inc., 1967), p. 51.
6. From *The Process of Communication: An Introduction to Theory and Practice,* by David Berlo, p. 72. Copyright © 1960 by Holt, Rinehart & Winston, Inc. Reprinted by permission of Holt, Rinehart & Winston.
7. See Eleanor C. Hein, *Communication in Nursing Practice* (Boston: Little, Brown, 1973).
8. Other models that have been developed include those by David Berlo, *The Process of Communication* (New York: Holt, Rinehart & Winston, 1960), p. 72; F. H. George, *Cybernetics and Biology* (San Francisco: W. H. Freeman & Company Publishers, 1965), p. 21; and C. E. Shannon and W. Weaver, *The Mathematical Theory of Communication* (Urbana, Ill.: University of Illinois Press, 1949), p. 98.

BIBLIOGRAPHY

Annett, John, *Feedback and Human Behavior.* Baltimore: Penguin Books, 1969.
Berlo, David, *The Process of Communication: An Introduction to Theory and Practice.* New York: Holt, Rinehart & Winston, 1960.
DeFleur, Melvin L. and Larsen, Otto N., *The Flow of Information: An Experiment in Mass Communication.* New York: Harper & Row, 1958.
George, F. H., *Cybernetics and Biology.* San Francisco: W. H. Freeman & Company, Publishers, 1965.
Hall, Edward T., *The Silent Language.* New York: Doubleday, 1959.
Harms, L. S., *Intercultural Communication.* New York: Harper & Row, 1973.
Hein, Eleanor C., *Communication in Nursing Practice.* Boston: Little, Brown, 1973.
Katz, Daniel, "Psychological Barriers to Communication," *The Annals of the Academy of Political and Social Science,* 250, (March 1947).
Reid, Clyde, *The Empty Pulpit.* New York: Harper & Row, 1967.
Samovar, Larry A. and Rintye, Edward D., "Interpersonal Communication: Some Working Principles," in *Small Group Communication: A Reader,* ed. Robert S. Cathcart and Larry A. Samovar. Dubuque, Ia.: W. C. Brown, 1970.
Schramm, Wilbur, "How Communication Works," in *The Process and Effects of Mass Communication,* ed. Wilbur Schramm. Urbana, Ill.: University of Illinois Press, 1955.

SHANNON, C. E., and WEAVER, W. *The Mathematical Theory of Communication.* Urbana, Ill.: University of Illinois Press, 1949.

WATZLAWICK, PAUL, BEAVIN, JANET HELMICK, and JACKSON, DON D., *Pragmatics of Human Communication.* New York: W. W. Norton & Co. Inc., 1967.

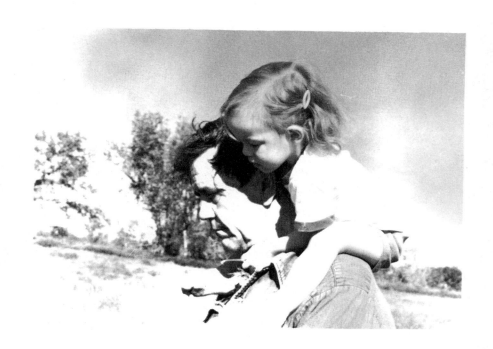

PERSONAL
ASPECTS OF
COMMUNICATION

II

*It has been generally agreed that true and
full human living is based on three
components: intrapersonal dynamics,
interpersonal relationships, and a
frame of reference.*

JOHN POWELL, S.J.*

41

KEY POINTS

CHAPTER 3
Definition of Perception
Perception of Self
ingredients of feeling good about
yourself
sources of self-perceptions
Perception of Others
selective perception
Personal Perception Choices
perception of self and others
demographic factors
psychological factors

CHAPTER 4
Definition of Roles
Factors Influencing Roles
assigned role expectation
chosen roles
patient feedback
dental context

CHAPTER 5
**Personal Aspects of Commu-
nication**
trust
emotion
reason
Verbal Communication
connotative meaning
denotative meaning
style
Vocal Communication
articulation
pronunciation
**Nonverbal-Nonvocal Commu-
nication**
body movements, facial
expressions distance, touch,
objects, odor, status, time,
dress and grooming

Perception

3

Reflect for a moment on the perceptions you have formed about places you have been, people you have met, food you have eaten, and the reactions you had to these and similar situations. Have you ever thought seriously about why you responded the way you did? Your responses were most likely based on your perceptions.

Definition of Perception

Perception is what an individual has experienced in his or her past which has caused a set of assumptions to develop. These assumptions are then used as guidelines to interpret the meaning of every subsequent experience in life. Brooks and Emmert further define perception as "a mental process in which we select, organize, and interpret the many stimuli that impinge on us at any given moment."[1] Actually, it is the assigning of meaning to sensory information. Thus, the formation of impressions is the way in which individuals view and evaluate each other in direct communication interaction. It is the process by which the body interprets and receives sensory input that establishes the basis for communication.

Perhaps you have had the experience of completely changing your initial thoughts about a person after you have come to know him or her over a longer period of time. This is an example of *changed perceptions*. The forma-

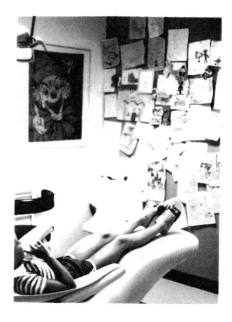

Figure 3-1. This young patient sitting in a dental operatory is interpreting and receiving many kinds of sensory input, which establishes the basis of her communication with the dental health team.

tion of your ideas about things, places, and people is of particular significance to you as a dental professional. The perception your patients have of you and vice versa is a vital factor in your interpersonal and professional communication with them.

Imagine you are with a friend and bump into an acquaintance who is with three of her friends in a restaurant in which you are all having dinner. Your conversation begins with the formal "Hello," and then your friend introduces you to her companions: "I would like you to meet Marge, Diane, and Pat. Marge and Diane teach English and Pat is Steve Balsiger's wife—you know, he's the quarterback for the Kansas City Chiefs!" What might be your impressions and initial thoughts about the three women? Would you be conscious of their responses to you? How would their professional roles affect your impression of them as individuals? Think for a moment about the three women and your perceptions of them.

Who would be most likely to impress you the most? Why? It is interesting that certain professions and positions influence a person's perceptions. A well-known football player's wife perhaps seems more interesting and "memorable" than a teacher. Perceptions of individuals' professional status and position play a significant role in our thoughts about and impressions of patients as health-care professionals.

Another example of the different ways in which we all perceive is the case of the dental hygienist who notes on a patient's record that he has had "good home-care procedures," also noting that bleeding points exist on teeth

#3, #4, #28 as well as periodontal readings of 5 mm on the same teeth. What does the dental hygienist perceive as "good home care" in her patient's oral cavity? From what point of comparison does the dental hygienist decide the patient has had "good" home-care techniques? What is "good" to one may be "bad" to another. Consider, as an illustration of the semantic problem in perception, all of the following meanings of the word "good":

morally righteous	honest
honorable	conscientious
behaviorally proper	suitable
useful	valuable
agreeable	satisfying
technically competent	reliable
healthy	appropriate
favorable	commendable
approvable	notable for achievement

Would any of these be more accurate than the word "good"? Or is "good" even the best word to use as a description on a dental record in the first place? A more quantitative description might be more accurate. Some authorities in periodontics say that any area of bleeding signifies disease and that a 5-mm pocket depth cannot be adequately cleaned and maintained with a toothbrush and floss.

PERCEPTION OF SELF

Probably life's greatest achievement is learning about yourself. How comfortable you are with yourself and others stems from your self-image. If you consciously think of yourself as an excellent dental auxiliary, then each time during the day when you achieve something good, your self-image as a professional is reinforced. When you recognize that it is good, this reinforces your self-image even more. Continually, during a productive day at the office, your subconscious mind is fed with good thoughts about your professionalism, and gradually they become true. Your creative self-consciousness then takes over so that you act like your new self-image. This process is commonly called the *self-fulfilling prophecy*. Your mind automatically provides you with the energy, creativity, and motivation needed to reach realistic goals you set for yourself in life.[2]

Consider your public and private roles, and the relationship they have to your behavior. What you want others to think of you in one place—in the dental office, for example— and who you are in your private life, are very significant elements in all your interpersonal communication experiences.

Psychologist John Powell, in his book *Fully Human, Fully Alive,* discusses five essential ingredients in feeling good about yourself. His five steps of achieving life to its fullest are: (1) to accept oneself, (2) to be oneself, (3) to forget oneself in loving, (4) to believe in something, and (5) to have a feeling of belonging.[3]

Your Self-Inventory

As you begin to think more specifically about your own concept of your role as a dental auxiliary, how do you perceive yourself? What qualities do you possess that are assets to your character? How will these qualities influence your performance as a dental assistant or dental hygienist? A self-inventory is presented in Communication Exercise 3-1. Forty traits are listed in the inventory. These are qualities or traits that we hear dental auxiliaries express during personal interviews. They are both positive as well as negative factors affecting the dependent variables of office productivity, professional staff satisfaction, and quality dental care in their particular team. Beside each quality are four columns labeled from left to right as follows: "I have most often . . . ," "I would like to be . . . more often," "I am least often . . . ," and "I would like to be . . .". For each of the items on the list, place a check mark on the line that best describes how you perceive yourself in situations in which you deal with other people. When you have finished the self-inventory, take a moment to reflect on how you feel about yourself as a future member of a dental health team. Do you feel good about yourself and the qualities that you checked? Or are there several qualities you believe you need to work more seriously on? Which qualities do you consider to be the most important when dealing with other people?

COMMUNICATION EXERCISE 3-1

Check each quality or trait in the column that most appropriately describes you from the list below.

	I AM MOST OFTEN . . .	I WOULD LIKE TO BE . . . MORE OFTEN	I AM LEAST OFTEN . . .	I WOULD LIKE TO BE . . .
1. Honest				
2. Genuine				
3. Accepting				
4. Supportive				
5. Concrete				
6. Compromising				

	I AM MOST OFTEN . . .	I WOULD LIKE TO BE . . . MORE OFTEN	I AM LEAST OFTEN . . .	I WOULD LIKE TO BE . . .
7. Initiative-taking				
8. Careful listening				
9. Sensitive				
10. Responsible				
11. Assertive				
12. Lazy				
13. Owner of my actions				
14. Honest about my inadequacies				
15. Flexible				
16. Willing to change				
17. Critical of others				
18. Empathetic				
19. A leader				
20. Sharing				
21. A grudge-holder				
22. An open communicator				
23. Defensive				
24. Respected by others				
25. Respectful of others				
26. Loyal				
27. Persevering				
28. Competent in technical skills				
29. Ethical				
30. Patient				
31. Self-confident				
32. Anxious				
33. Ambitious				
34. Humorous				
35. Willing to deal with problems immediately				
36. Tolerant				
37. Self-respecting				
38. Stubborn				
39. Persuasive				
40. Friendly				

To a large extent, your feeling good about yourself or not so good about yourself as a dental auxiliary will reflect on how you engage in your professional responsibilities in a dental office, deal with patients, and communicate with your peers. The purpose of the self-inventory is to illustrate that the way you feel about yourself and how you perceive your personal and professional worth will probably influence your performance and interpersonal relationships on a dental health team. Your perception of those you work with and the way you treat them will depend on how you feel about yourself. If there are qualities that are negative, that do not please you, then begin now to devise a plan for improvement in those areas. If we could see ourselves as others see us, most of us would instinctively spend less time worrying and procrastinating and get busy improving ourselves.

Try to look at yourself through the eyes of those with whom you work or with whom you have daily interactions. Have someone else rate you according to the forty qualities listed in Communication Exercise 3–1. How does your own self-rating compare to that person's rating of you? What qualities are different? Why? What similarities do you find? Are you perceived by others as possessing qualities that would be positive factors on a dental health team?

Developing methods of self-improvement and self-acceptance are key factors in your success as a dental professional with patients, as well as with peers. They are also essential ingredients in establishing contentment in your personal life. In his book, Powell notes that to feel good about yourself you have to learn to love. That is a powerful statement—one that may not seem appropriate to discuss in this text on communication skills for dental auxiliaries. But personal experiences have proven to many of us that the feeling of loving and being loved by our families, friends, and spouses helps to create within us a feeling of self-worth. Without this feeling, developing a sense of self-acceptance will be a difficult challenge in any facet of life, including your daily work.

Looking at the traits which you identify as your own, ask yourself, "How do I feel about being who I am?" Some days may find you feeling good about yourself and on other days you may not feel so good. Communication with others is influenced by how you, the source of your own messages and the receiver of others' messages, behave each day.

Self-Acceptance

But how do you accept yourself? Where does self-image originate? Why does it constantly fluctuate? Social scientists contend that the process of developing one's self-perceptions involves a variety of factors. Some of these include (1) the pursuit of self-esteem, (2) the approval of others and their evaluative reactions, (3) personal expectations, (4) identification with role models, (5) roles played, (6) masks worn in and for certain occasions, and (7) identity formation beginning in adolescence. [4] Let us investigate some of these factors in more detail.

APPROVAL OF OTHERS.   As the dental hygienist prepares to polish her patient's teeth, the patient says to her, "You are so gentle when you clean my teeth, I have never had my teeth cleaned so thoroughly before." Or, a dentist tells his dental assistant after a busy day in the office, "You always know what I need ahead of time." These positive compliments from the patient and dentist should create a good feeling about your professional self-image. Remember the importance you placed on your parents' responses to you when you were a child. Think of how their reactions to you affected your self-image.

IDENTITY FORMATION.   One woman grew up believing she was ugly. Her parents' attitude and behavior toward her, as a young person with a cosmetic facial scar and speech defect, implied that she was deformed, stupid, and ugly. Therefore, as a child, she adopted her parents' image and comments as true. She had no reason to believe otherwise; so, for years she truly believed she *was* ugly, deformed, and stupid. Self-concept is developed, in part, as a result of what we learn about ourselves from other significant people in our lives.

ROLE PLAYING.   How many dozens of times have you compared yourself to your classmates? Or the competitor ahead of you in an athletic event? It seems to be human nature for everyone to compare themselves and their personal worth and abilities with other individuals who display similar qualities, expertise, and desires. To imitate others is another way some people choose to form a self-image. This is called "role playing."

ROLE TAKING.   Another aspect of developing self-concept is role *taking*—choosing to take roles such as the role of a dental auxiliary. As you go through dental hygiene or dental assisting school you will consider yourself as a "dental hygienist" or "dental assistant" for a variety of reasons. Often you may see yourself primarily in the terms of a job you perform or the career you have chosen. As a student you play a certain role and as a professional dental auxiliary you play yet another role when you are with patients. In what ways does your role as a professional affect your personal self-perception?

ROLE MODELS.   While you are in training, many people will influence you in a multitude of ways. Possibly, someone has already played a role in your life because you have chosen a career as a certified dental assistant or as a dental hygienist. That someone with whom you have identified is a *model*. He or she has been significant in establishing a portion of your professional self-identity. Possibly, it is the way this person dresses and behaves that makes you want to dress and act in a similar manner. Our values and actions are greatly influenced by our role models.

CAREER CHOICE.   Usually during late adolescence, individuals are forced to decide about all the pieces of self-identity that they can take hold of and cultivate. Think about why you have decided to become a dental hygienist or dental assistant. What qualities do you possess that have made you want to serve humankind? How do you know you have these qualities? Perhaps someone in high school said to you that you had good dexterity and should consider a career in dentistry. Possibly you did volunteer work and gained great personal satisfaction from helping other people. Adolescence is a very impressionable time in our lives, and the factors influencing us are often critical in determining the direction we take in career pursuits.

PERCEPTION OF OTHERS

How do our own perceptions of ourselves color our all-important perceptions of others? And how does the way we "see" others influence our effectiveness as dental professionals?

Imagine that a new patient has just come into the office for dental treatment. The normal procedure for the dental auxiliary is to gather a medical history and make an initial examination of the patient's head, neck, and oral structures. This is followed by an oral prophylaxis including the removal of all soft and hard deposits, polishing of the teeth and restorations, patient education, charting of defective restorations and periodontal disease, and a full series of radiographs. The dentist then proceeds with the diagnosis and treatment planning. In the process of the dental hygienist's examination and prophylaxis, suppose our hypothetical patient responds very negatively, saying that his last dentist did not waste time cleaning teeth and taking X-rays, and he did not think it was necessary now.

Think about this new patient. He is expressing that he does not need his teeth cleaned or X-rayed because the last dentist he went to did not think such procedures were necessary. Why? Was it painful? Maybe the expense is of concern to him. Consider what you are thinking about him. How are you responding to his comments? Are you remembering the last patient who talked like this to you? Remember that both of you are forming perceptions of each other.

If your initial impressions and assessments of new patients are based on solid and thoughtful reasoning, based on past experience and empathy, more effective communication can occur. On the other hand, if your perceptions are not accurate, communication difficulties may develop, hindering good communication and effective dental treatment. Thus, for a dental auxiliary, the first encounter with a patient is of vital importance. It is this initial time in which perceptions and judgments are made by both you and the patient. Based on this initial contact, the communication process throughout the entire dental visit is established.

Selective Perception

In everyday professional and personal–interpersonal communication encounters, a barrier to successful experiences is the tendency for most of us to see only what we want to see, hear only what we want to hear, and believe only what we want to believe. Probably the rationale for this selective perception is our interest in controlling the predictability of our relationships. Intentional and nonintentional expectations of people and things narrow our perception and tend to make us see only what we want to see, evaluate, and believe. *Selective perception* refers to the phenomenon of assigning meaning to all the various messages transmitted and received by another person. In order to interpret these messages, we depend upon our past experiences.

For example, a small boy, Bill, was seated in the dental chair for his monthly fluoride treatment. A white-uniformed stranger—one who seemed unfriendly and who spoke in a rough voice—entered the room. He had never seen her before and she acted quite gruff toward him. Bill really did not know what was going on. He had always been fearful of his dental visits anyway, but this really made him anxious. On every other visit, the dentist himself had given Bill his fluoride treatment. So the new person in the office was a total surprise to him. When she began her examination of him, he began to cough because of a tickle in his throat. The woman said rather sharply, "Bill, don't cough! I'm trying to work on you. You're not being cooperative." As she became more stern with him, his perception of her became even more negative. Later, when he asked who she was, he was told that she was "the dental hygienist." From that point on, anyone who bore the label "dental hygienist" was perceived as being a stern, insensitive, gruff, unfriendly person.

Selective perception goes beyond routine perception. It narrows the scope of one's acceptance of others. In Bill's case, his perception of dental hygienists was firmly set by his first experience. Because this experience was reinforced by regular visits to the same dental office, the narrow perception had no reason to change. As a teenager, this boy changed dentists but retained his perception of "hygienists." He preferred to avoid them. His perception had become "selective." Selective perception, then, is seeing and hearing only what you want to see and hear while not fully understanding the other person's situation.

Basically then, as a result of our life experiences in general, we learn to perceive in particular ways. We perceive what we think other people are transmitting to us. Likewise, we have perceptions of the people with whom we are communicating. It is important to know about this basic phenomenon in learning how to be most effective as a dental professional. The patient's response to the procedures in the dental office is important. And so are the dental hygienist's or dental assistant's perceptions and impressions of the patient. If we have limited selective perception, we perceive what we expect and want to perceive because our past interpretations of experiences have made us assume that these expectations are true. Such a narrow view can only limit our effectiveness.

PERSONAL PERCEPTION CHOICES

Having considered your perceptions of yourself and of others, and having reflected on how these perceptions have developed, let us discuss the basis for your personal perception choices. How you perceive yourself affects your perception of others, and because of mutual feedback, each person's perception affects the communication process as it develops. In general terms, there are three types of perceptions you can have about yourself and about the other person: (1) positive, (2) neutral, and (3) negative.

Positive Perceptions	Those which make you feel good about yourself and others, usually allowing open and nonjudgmental communication to occur.
Neutral Perceptions	Those which involve no strong assumptions or expectations for either you or the person to live up to or to achieve.
Negative Perceptions	Those which cause you to feel inadequate, unimportant, incompetent, or less worthy than others; or those which cause you to have similar judgments about others, causing you to "put them down."

COMMUNICATION EXERCISE 3-2

Complete the following statements. Put them away for a few days and then look at them when you have time to conscientiously reflect upon the perceptions and beliefs you have about yourself. From what different sources do you think you have developed these perceptions about yourself? How do they influence your perceptions of your peers, or of the patients who come into your office? Are they neutral, positive, or negative perceptions? What kind of perceptions do they elicit about other individuals—positive, negative or neutral?

My strongest personal conviction concerns . . .
I love . . .
When I meet someone for the first time I . . .
I feel most affectionate when . . .
I am happiest when . . .
I am afraid of . . .
I believe professionally in . . .
My weakest point is . . .
I feel jealous when . . .
I feel ashamed when . . .
My greatest asset is . . .
I am a good . . .
I expect personally to . . .
I expect professionally to . . .
I feel adequate when . . .
I am irritated the most by . . .
I should always . . .
My role in preventive dentistry is . . .
I am . . .

Factors Affecting Personal Perceptions

When a patient enters the dental office, impressions and assumptions are formulated almost instantaneously as a result of the immediate environment that is presented. The first person to greet the patient is the receptionist or business manager, and as the interpersonal communication continues to develop between the patient and that person, initial feelings are reinforced, intensified, and altered. Also, entirely new perceptions may be introduced and the structure of perceptions becomes more and more complex.

Therefore, it is important to be conscious of how you determine the perceptions that you create about and in the patients who enter the dental office. Some demographic factors that affect perception include (1) sex, (2) age, (3) race, (4) religion, and (5) beliefs. In addition, an individual's perceptions are also influenced by psychological factors such as (1) attitudes and emotions, (2) values, (3) culture, (4) roles, and (5) societal demands. As Figure 3–2 illustrates, there are many avenues individuals use in "choosing" perceptions from their previous expectations and assumptions. Following are some

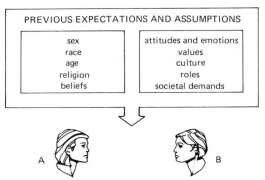

Figure 3-2. Sources of perception.

real-life examples of how these factors affect personal perception choices within the dental setting.

SEX.   One's gender can affect perceptions. A man seeking dental care entered a large university dental clinic. Very indignantly he said, "I do not want to be assigned to a woman dental student for my new crown." When asked why, he replied, "I do not want a women to see how bad my mouth looks." Apparently, his comments reflected his social desire not to weaken his masculine image because he valued a woman's perception of him.

AGE.   A 24-year-old dental hygienist was hired to work in a new dental office. After a few days, during a conversation with her dentist, she commented on the difficulty she was having in getting along with one of the dental assistants. "I think the problem stems from the fact that we just do not have anything in common. She is only 19 years old!" Age was negatively influencing the dental hygienist's perception of the dental assistant.

RACE.   A white patient was admitted to a Midwestern dental-school pain clinic. At that particular time, the only dentist available to treat the patient was black. The patient vehemently told the dental assistant that she did not want to be treated by a black dentist. However, since he was the only clinician available to treat her pain, she had no choice but to receive his treatment. Afterwards, she asked if she could be assigned to him for additional dental treatment. Obviously, the patient's initial perception was influenced by his race. Happily, this perception changed after she got to know him and could alter her perception.

RELIGION.   One patient presented a dental hygienist with a book entitled *God Can Fill Teeth*. The dental hygienist thought to herself, "This lady is a real religious nut! I'll just get her teeth cleaned as quickly as I can and get her out." Could the book alone influence the hygienist's perception of this particular patient? Perhaps the hygienist's initial perceptions were reinforced by some other things done by the patient, such as rather obviously praying, or trying to convert patients in the waiting room.

The important thing to remember from this example is that health professionals must be conscious of their perceptions of patients, because every individual entering into their operatory deserves the same high-quality preventive treatment the last patient received, no matter how the patient is perceived personally. Individual perceptions can cause distractions away from the real purpose of the appointment, causing a professional to render less than quality preventive care to all patients.

Emotional Factors

As people experience the many sensory stimuli affecting their daily lives, they automatically respond with emotions. Attitudinal and emotional factors influence a person's perceptions of everything in the environment, including patients. For example, reflect back to the patient who said he did not think getting his teeth cleaned and having radiographs were necessary because the last dentist had not thought it was important. By the time this patient was seated in the dental chair it was 4:30 P.M. Already during the day, the dental hygienist had had to deal with a flat tire on the way to work, an insufficient check, and a full set of blank radiographs because of a malfunctioning machine. This patient with his complaint was the last thing she needed to be dealing with in one day. So she threw up her arms in distress and let the dentist handle the situation.

VALUES.   In a society in which a new freedom and more liberal standard of morality is flourishing, the question of values may be significantly different for the generation of people who grew up in the '30s, compared to the generation who grew up in the '60s. The important thing to remember is that being aware of and sensitive to differing values is essential when dealing with patients of varying ages and moral standards. For example, many people who grew up in the depression years of the 1930s went to the dentist only out of necessity. Money was very tight, and a person usually visited the dentist to get teeth pulled or fixed. Today, however, young people are visiting the dentist on a regular basis to learn how to take care of their teeth, not necessarily to get them fixed. The same holds true for patients that are on three-month recalls because they want the dental hygienist to clean their teeth. They may not place a high value on daily brushing and flossing for preventive purposes. Primarily, they may be brushing for cosmetic reasons only.

Through our many life experiences, each of us has developed a certain set of values by which we live. These have been formed from a variety of sources. Two factors that should be understood are socialization messages and the "better-than" messages we received in our childhood from parents, teachers, and other role models. The following are some socialization messages you may have received. They may have been verbal as well as nonverbal messages.

> "Children should be seen and not heard."
> "If you can't say anything nice, don't say anything at all."
> "Don't talk with your mouth full of food."
> "Don't rock the boat or make waves."
> "It is as important to be a good loser as to be a good winner."
> "You chose to do it—now you must take the consequences."

Or consider the "better-than" messages that may have influenced you during your childhood:

> "Men are stronger than women."
> "Formal education is better than learned trade skills."
> "Women are better cooks than men."
> "A medical degree is better than a Ph.D."

The demographic factors of race, sex, age, and religion have been important in the establishment of our values in the "better-than" messages we have received. Reflect for a moment on these two kinds of messages. Values do play an important role in our perceptions of other people, but they are also difficult to definitively substantiate and discuss.

Carl Rogers' studies of attitudes give an insight into the best ways to perceive others' value systems. Two significant points Rogers makes relating to a therapist's relationship with patients can be realistically compared to the helping relationship most dental auxiliaries experience:

1. Procedures and techniques are less important than a professional's attitudes about the patient and situation.
2. It is the manner in which a professional's attitudes and procedures are perceived by a patient that is crucial. [5]

Consider how you developed your attitudes about dentistry and becoming a dental auxiliary. Your attitude about people and the work that you do relates directly to your value system, which was influenced by many socialization and "better-than" messages from a variety of demographic sources. Communication Exercises 3–3 and 3–4 will help you understand more about value formation.

COMMUNICATION EXERCISE 3–3

List some socialization messages you received as a child.

1.

2.

3.

4.

Think about the "better-than" messages you received. List them below.

1.

2.

3.

4.

Express how these affect your communication with friends, family, peers, and patients. Do they bring to mind specific values that you hold about yourself and your life?

COMMUNICATION EXERCISE 3–4

Milton Rokeach, from the University of Western Ontario, developed a values survey in 1966 as a major portion of a research project. In the following exercise, which is similar to that used by Rokeach,[6] rank the following values in descending order from what you consider to be the most important value (number 1) to what you consider the least important value (number 18). While you rank the values, cover up the results of the survey, below, that was given to two groups of dental professionals.

RANK	VALUE
_____	A comfortable life
_____	An exciting life
_____	A sense of accomplishment
_____	A world at peace
_____	A world of beauty
_____	Equality
_____	Family security

(continued)

COMMUNICATION EXERCISE 3-4 (*Contd*)

RANK	VALUE
_____	Freedom
_____	Happiness
_____	Inner harmony
_____	Mature love
_____	National security
_____	Pleasure
_____	Salvation
_____	Social recognition
_____	Self-respect
_____	True friendship
_____	Wisdom

You will find at the end of this chapter the results of this survey as it was given to 7 dental hygiene faculty members and 44 dental hygiene students in May 1976 at the University of Missouri–Kansas City, School of Dentistry.[7]

GUIDELINES FOR UNDERSTANDING OTHERS' VALUES.   When you meet a patient for the first time, remember that you do not know what specific set of values he or she lives by in daily life. But the person's value system will indeed affect his or her perception of you as a dental auxiliary, and in turn, your values will affect your perception of the patient. Because of the attitudes and beliefs that make up our value system, it is vitally important to be aware of and responsive to them as we make perceptions of other people. In any interpersonal encounter, whether it be in the dental setting or socially, keep in mind the following suggestions when establishing your perception of another individual:

1. Remember that the values most important to you and those that you think are relevant will affect your perceptions significantly. For example, the patient who will not floss his teeth even with the knowledge of the periodontal consequences may be perceived as uncooperative and disinterested. Such a perception may be formed because you, the dental auxiliary, believe it to be a priority in daily hygiene routines. The patient, in turn, may be a 70-year-old thinking, "Who does this young lady think she *is*, telling me to floss my teeth every morning?"

2. Often, the importance you place on some attitudes and beliefs makes you ignore certain characteristics, cues, or talents of another individual. It is important to keep an open mind about others. In dental assisting school and dental hygiene school, young professionals are introduced to a particular

code for their respective professions. The code establishes guidelines for dress, conduct, and attitude appropriate for health settings. A dental assistant confided in one of the authors concerning her disapproval of the other assistant; she thought that person "looked like a slob." The one about whom she was talking wore blue jeans, nail polish, and dangling earrings. It is significant that, despite her somewhat unorthodox appearance, the dentist would not fire her; he obviously thought she had potential and worth in his practice. He was able to see other traits which were not filtered out by his own value system.

3. Many people tend to avoid information, things, people, and places that are inconsistent with their values and beliefs. It is very natural for us to want to associate with others who have similar backgrounds, education, and thoughts about their profession. We may seek people and information that enhances our own value system and causes us to believe that it is acceptable to others. But such selective attention should be avoided, because it can cause us to ignore the validity of other information and lifestyles.

4. One way to overcome perceptions based only on your own value system is to try to walk in the other person's shoes before passing judgment. A young patient, 8 years old, was creating quite a scene in the dentist's chair. She was screaming and crying as the dental hygienist tried to take bitewings. Needless to say, this behavior didn't encourage positive perceptions on the part of the office staff. When the patient returned a year later for her recall appointment, the attitude of the staff was, "Guess what little brat we have to contend with today!" Later, the dentist learned that this little girl had been submitted to child abuse; her response in the office was likely from fear of pain and suffering. When they learned this, the staff members changed their perceptions.

CULTURAL INFLUENCE.   The culture in which a person lives definitely plays a role in developing perceptual impressions. Everyone is significantly influenced by an array of ever-present traditions, role expectations, norms, models, and values; and these differ for every cultural background. For example, the *right time* and the *correct amount of time* are relative factors depending upon a particular culture's perspective of time. In Germany, being prompt is very important. When you are invited to a cocktail party at 8:00 P.M., you are expected to be there at 8:00 P.M. In the United States, however, being on time to an 8:00 P.M. cocktail party is for many "bad form."

One cultural perception concerning time that affects health professionals is the scheduling and maintaining of appointments with patients. Most of us are punctual for dental and medical appointments because we know the doctor's time is as important as our own. However, in some cultures, to be expected to arrive promptly is considered a personal and professional insult.

It may imply that you are not very busy and thereby not very important if you can arrange your schedule to be prompt for appointments. Culture also helps to determine a person's perception and interpretation of health and sickness. Thus, an understanding of a patient's or peer's culture and its relevance in his or her life is vitally important when establishing effective interpersonal communication.

ROLES.   How do people let roles of others affect their perceptions? Consider this: When someone asks, "What do you do?" and you answer, "I'm a dental assistant," an example of a negative response from that person might be, "How can you stand to look in dirty mouths all day long?" The point of this example is that the roles people have in life influence others' perceptions of them. Being a dental assistant does not necessarily mean you work in mouths all day long. If you had stated that you taught dental auxiliary utilization at the university dental school, a totally different response and impression might have been created. You would have had a different "role" in that person's eyes.

SOCIETAL DEMANDS.   Finally, the demands of society influence our personal perception choices. Mass media advertising indicates in a variety of ways the idea that, for white females, being slender and tan is synonymous with being beautiful. Thus, those who are not white, slender, and tan may find it difficult to prove to others (or to believe) that they are truly beautiful in their own way. Why? Because our society has placed significance on looking like models in magazine ads. This, in turn, may affect how others perceive us and how we perceive ourselves as important persons.

As you have read through this section, you should now be aware of the many influential factors that affect your perceptual choices. The point to remember, however, is that you can choose your perceptions so that they work with you and not against you during interpersonal communication encounters in the dental auxiliary field.

SUMMARY

It is evident that the process of perception is an extremely complex, eclectic, interrelated composition of a variety of communication processes. Perception is the process by which individuals sort the sensory stimuli from past experiences into assumptions and impressions that are transferable to present and future communication situations. Perceptions are not necessarily constant; they can be and often are changed. Our discussion has focused on the five ingredients to developing a good self-image: accepting oneself, being oneself, forgetting oneself in loving, believing in something, and having the feeling of belonging. We also investigated the six sources from which our personal perceptions stem: reactions of others, comparison of oneself to others, roles one plays, indentification of oneself with models, adolescent identity crises, and need for self-esteem. A person's perception of another is often related to his or her own perception of himself. It is important to remember however, that a person's perception of another greatly influences his or her own interpersonal communication choices. Selective perception refers to the way we establish meaning for all the varied messages transmitted and received by another individual. In many instances, it is based upon a person's past impressions and assumptions. Individuals choose to make perceptions and impressions based on a multitude of factors, including sex, age, race, religion, beliefs, attitudes and emotions, values, culture, roles, and societal demands.

Results of Values Survey

The most important values for the dental hygiene faculty were, respectively: inner harmony, self-respect, family security, mature love, and happiness.

The least important values for the dental hygiene faculty were, respectively: national security, salvation, an exciting life, pleasure, and a world at peace.

The most important values for dental hygiene students were, respectively: happiness, inner harmony, family security, mature love, and self-respect.

The least important values for dental hygiene students were, respectively: national security, equality, a world of beauty, a world at peace, and salvation.

CHAPTER ACTIVITIES

1. Write a definition of "perception" which includes the factors that affect your own perception of others in your personal, social, and professional life.
2. Write a description of the "ideal" dental patient. Once you have done this, list all the demographic factors that might conceivably affect your idea of the "ideal" person.
3. Compile a list of attributes you like about yourself. Next, underline those traits which you believe are helpful to a person in your chosen dental profession.
4. From the point of view of a dental patient, what do you think is a complete description of an ideal dental assistant? Of an ideal dental hygienist? Write brief descriptions similar to that in Activity 2 above.
5. Based on your experience with people, prepare a list of character traits that

give a negative "first impression" and that could thereby adversely affect the ease with which you can communicate with a person who has such traits.

6. Once you have done Activity 5, reflect on what would be required of you in order to overcome "first-impression" perceptions so as to work comfortably and most effectively with a patient in a dental situation. Discuss this with a classmate or associate.

REFERENCES

* Reprinted from *Fully Human, Fully Alive* by John Powell, S. J., © 1969 Argus Communications, Niles, Ill. Used with permission.

1. William O. Brooks and Phillip Emmert, *Interpersonal Communication*, 2nd ed. (Dubuque, Ia.: W. C. Brown, 1976), p. 86.

2. Additional reading on this subject can be found in Rudolph F. Verderber and Kathleen S. Verderber, *Inter-Act Using Communication Skills*, 2nd ed. (Belmont, Cal.: Wadsworth, 1980), p. 35.

3. Powell, *Fully Human, Fully Alive*, p. 23.

4. Carl Rogers, "The Characteristics of a Helping Relationship" (paper delivered at the APGA Convention, St. Louis, Mo., March 31–April 3, 1958).

5. Ibid.

6. Milton Rokeach, "Long Range Experimental Modifications of Values, Attitudes, and Behavior" (paper presented as part of a symposium, *Human Behavior and its Control*, American Association for the Advancement of Science, Chicago, Ill., 1970).

7. Joseph S. Sakumura, "Values of Dental Hygiene Faculty and Students," *Educational Directions*, 2, no. 2, (May 1977), 6–8.

Role Behavior in the Dental Environment

4

In this chapter we discuss the roles of dental auxiliaries and the roles of patients in preventive dental care. The roles of other professionals on the dental health team are important, too, and will be dealt with in Part IV. This chapter concentrates on the dental auxiliary and the patient in terms of a particular interpersonal communication dyad.

Remember in the last chapter, we said that you have choices to make about your perceptions. You have a choice to make about how you perceive yourself—as a private person, a social person, and a professional person. You also must make choices about your perceptions of patients—as individuals from diverse backgrounds, as individuals with unique needs and emotions, and as persons seeking a special kind of care from you—namely, preventive dental care. As you develop these choices about your perceptions of yourself and others, you also develop the foundation of your professional role.

Definition of Role

A person's role is his or her function or identity related to a task or responsibility. Sometimes our perception of ourselves influences the roles we have. Other times, our roles influence our perceptions as well as the perceptions others have of us. Hence, perceptions and roles are very closely related.

For the purposes of this discussion, a role is defined as the various interpersonal and technical functions a person performs in the dental office. It is a set of perceptions that a person has as to how he or she should act and perform on a dental health team. It also includes the perception of the behavior of other team members in a dental environment. The role a person plays is, in part, determined by the individual's self-perception and expectations in one's personal frame of reference. Hence, perceptions and roles are very closely related.

FACTORS INFLUENCING ROLES

We develop roles to match generally accepted cultural expectations and thereby to "fit in" with those around us. Each culture has its own expectations of people. Each smaller group within a large culture usually has its own special expectations. For example, in white middle-class Midwestern America, overt displays of emotion may not seem "appropriate" during daily activities such as shopping and casual conversation. Yet the same people in this cultural group may scream and shout uncontrollably at a hotly contested basketball game in the high school gymnasium. Roles change according to circumstances and expectations. If you were to scream and shout with excitement while shopping each time you see a food item you like, yet sit silently and expressionless at an exciting ball game, your role in each situation would be considered inappropriate.

CULTURAL ROLES.   Conformity to role expectations is learned as we live in our society. Moving from region to region or traveling from country to country may cause temporary confusion until the traveler learns what is generally expected in behavior roles.

Deviance from cultural expectations is often judged as "bad" and may even carry moral implications. In large metropolitan areas in some regions of America, it may be appropriate for a shopper at a bargain sale to push and shove and snatch the items most desired. In smaller towns, such role behavior by a shopper might be inappropriate, and likely to be considered rude and inconsiderate.

SOCIAL ROLES.   Beyond such public forms of role behavior, you have social roles in various aspects of life. At a party of friends whom you know, you are likely to take on the role that you have found fits your relationship with them. You may be the "jolly one" or the "intellectual one" or the "religious one." When you choose to conform to one behavior regularly, which others grow to expect, a role is established.

FAMILY ROLES.   Roles are most easily seen in families. In a family, each person has a role which others learn to take for granted. Although many roles are changing in the traditional family, with some roles being shared, each person usually assumes some role that is important to the smooth functioning of the family unit. One person may be the person who fixes things, while another may be the primary parent, taking responsibility for the children. Each child also may have an identifiable role, based on his or her interests or the parent's expectations. Parents may be able to end children's disputes, for example, because the adults may choose to undertake the role of "dispute-settlers." One parent may have the role of setting up social engagements for the family, while the other may be the one to take care of major financial decisions. When each person knows the roles which they and the others play, there is predictability. Predictability in human relationships reduces the need to check constantly on what the other is doing to make the group life run well. Some roles, of course, can be damaging to the one who has them. The role of the "dumb kid" can be carried to the extreme if it causes a child to lose self-confidence and develop low self-esteem. Being sick in order to gain attention can develop into a role of childlike dependence. Roles guide behavior and bring about expectations from others. When a person decides to change or alter a role, especially in a family, it may cause confusion and disruption—as often occurs when children grow up and take on identities that may not be compatible with what the parents have been used to.

WORK ROLES.   In another context, roles exist in work situations. The owner of a business may take on a "patriarchal" role, running the business as if it were a family and he were the "Father" with all power and wisdom. In such a case, the owner may place employees in childlike roles. They may not be able to make useful suggestions or to question the decisions made by the owner. On the other hand, if a boss sees his or her role as a manager of a system, the boss may be more open to suggestions for making the business run more smoothly, and less threatened by employee suggestions. As with roles in family and social situations, roles at work result in a predictable group behavior. If the role is changed, there can be confusion and disruption of the system. People will not know how to communicate with the person with the changed role, at least temporarily. If, for example, an assembly-line worker is promoted to supervisor, other assembly-line workers, who used to be that person's friends, may now approach the new supervisor to express a complaint in different ways than they would have shared the same information before. Words may be more carefully selected; facial expressions and other nonverbal displays of feeling may be different than before. And, because the new supervisor may feel that he (or she) has more power, he may begin to speak with more confidence, be more forceful, and become more assertive.

That person's self-perception and the perception of former peers may affect his behavior, primarily in his verbal and nonverbal communication behavior. Work roles are not only determined by the task itself. They are also determined by the perceptions each person has of himself and the others around him. Away from the place of work, the roles may shift again, according to circumstances, tasks, and self-perceptions.

Emotional Attachment to Roles

Emotional attachment to roles is often strong. Consider your own expectations of how a child should and should not speak to a school teacher. You might expect the child to play the passive student role, one that keeps the child quiet and the teacher talking. Or you might expect the child to play a more active, assertive, participant role, asking the teacher questions and taking charge of his or her own learning. If you see a child verbally challenge a teacher, this may or may not fit your role expectation. And further, if the teacher becomes passive or submissive and does whatever the child says, you may feel that that is not the appropriate teacher's role. Ask yourself where your role expectations of students and teachers come from? Chances are, if you think back to your own childhood days in school, you may discover that your role expectations stem directly from the roles you took on when you were younger. It is not uncommon for adult parents who go to their child's school for a parent orientation meeting to sit passively in the small classroom chairs and raise their hand to speak, even though the teacher may be the same age or younger. Role expectations can become deeply embedded.

When others' role expectations of us do not fit our own image, emotional reactions can occur. If, in dental school, you are shown role models that fit your ideal of what a dental assistant or a dental hygienist should be, you may choose to talk and act in ways that fit that model. Once you go into a private office or clinic, you may find that patients, dentists, and other dental auxiliaries may not have the same "ideal" in their mind. If they remind you frequently that you are not conforming to their expectations, this may become a conflict for you and could affect your relationship with them. It is rarely an objective matter; emotional feelings are usually attached to roles.

Four situations generally influence the roles of dental assistants and dental hygienists. They are situations in which roles are (1) assigned, (2) chosen, and situations in which (3) patient feedback and (4) the dental context play a part.

Assigned Role Expectations

Assigned roles are those given to us. Sometimes they are defined in terms of broad social assumptions, sometimes in terms of specific task assignments. In terms of tasks, a dental auxiliary's role in the United States is specifically defined by rules and regulations established by individual state dental boards. Thus, much of your assigned role is defined, to a great extent, by the state in which you practice preventive dental care. For example, a dental hygienist who has graduated from an accredited dental hygiene program in certain states can administer local infiltration anesthesia; perform soft tissue currettage; place, condense, and carve restorations; and perform traditional roles defined by the profession, such as scaling subgingivally and supragingivally and polishing. Dental assistants, if certified, in certain states also can place, condense, and carve restorations, develop radiographs, take alginate impressions, and pour diagnostic study casts as well as performing traditionally assigned roles in assisting a dentist. Thus, in a dental office or clinic, titles often indicate assigned roles—namely, those associated with "RDH," "CDA," and "DDS," which appear on familiar name tags and framed certificates. These labels go with the assigned role and serve as general—though sometimes misunderstood—descriptions of what you do. They define the assigned role in that particular place.

Assigned roles and perceptions interact in a variety of ways. How you perceive your role and how a patient perceives your role may not be congruent. This divergence of perceptions can lead to communication difficulties. But these assigned roles are basically defined by your technical tasks and skills. Your skills are dependent on your knowledge and training in dental procedures. Beyond this, there remain three additional factors which influence your total identity.

Chosen Roles

Chosen roles add another dimension to your work. These are the behavioral and attitudinal attributes which set the pattern for what you do in addition to your technical responsibilities. These depend on how *you* chose to behave in relation to your patient and the attitude you have toward all that you do.

Chosen roles may be imitations of roles you see other people, whom you admire, act out. This "role-taking" manner of choosing roles may occur when there is some uncertainty, at first, about what behavior is appropriate to a particular situation or responsibility. If you have never been among dental professionals, but suddenly, in school, become acquainted with several persons in this field, you may well try to sort out those whom you admire from those who do not seem to be the kind of people who impress you in a positive way. Again, your perceptions are important. Because you have had little experience yourself in a dental role, yet find yourself becoming a dental auxiliary, it would not be unusual for you to try to imitate some of the role behaviors which you see in significant others in your field. As you take on others' role behaviors—including the areas of dress, grooming, attitude, speech patterns, and mannerisms—you are "testing" them or "trying them on

COMMUNICATION EXERCISE 4-1

Look over the list of behavioral and attitudinal terms listed below and check the column which you believe applies to your chosen profession.

BEHAVIOR OR ATTITUDE	ESSENTIAL TO YOUR EFFECTIVENESS	DESIRABLE	A "PLUS" BUT NOT ESSENTIAL	UNIMPORTANT OR NOT DESIRABLE
Outgoing				
Relaxed				
Gentle				
Good Listener				
Good Conversationalist				
Friendly				
Objective				
Sense of Humor				
Serious & Intent				
Empathetic/Caring				
Facially Expressionless				
Facially Expressive				
Emotionally Uninvolved				

Filling in this chart may give you an initial look at your own chosen role. Often, persons in health professions see themselves as "helping and caring people." These are subjective terms and have different connotations to different people. Still, they are important in defining your chosen role.

for size," so to speak. What seems to fit you will be retained and what seems uncomfortable, like clothing, will be rejected. Eventually, you may discover your own unique choices for role behavior and discard most of the behaviors which you have been acting out. This transition may come early in your career. Or it may take a while, as you move from place to place. As with your assigned role, your chosen role will affect your communication with patients and, in turn, affect your work.

Patient Feedback

There is a third influence on your total role identity. This is the *feedback* principle described in the first two chapters. Feedback, you may recall, serves to help you know how to adjust a communication behavior. The various ways in which a patient responds to you is feedback that may cause you to adjust your role behavior. For example, you may want to be conversational at the beginning of a dental appointment in order to establish rapport and put the patient at ease. The patient may not be interested in conversation, may send you a strong nonverbal message by giving you "silent" feedback, and may expect you simply to clean his teeth so he can leave. The more frequently you encounter this sort of feedback from a patient, the more sure you will be concerning your role in relationship to this particular patient.

The importance of this feedback in determining role behavior should not be overlooked. Watzlawick, Beavin, and Jackson emphasize the importance of both positive and negative feedback, noting that all interpersonal systems may be viewed as "feedback loops" because the behavior of each person affects the behavior of the other.[1]

Thus, the way you perceive the patient and the way you respond to patient *feedback* will affect your role behavior. If, for example, you see your role as one of a helping person with responsibility to make certain that every patient learns and practices "correct" preventive dental procedures, you likely will be more than a technician going to work for a daily paycheck. Rather, you might take on the additional roles of teacher, motivator, and persuader. If you see the patient's role as being a passive one, you could easily become impatient and defensive if the patient challenges your decisions. Negative feedback can alter your role, or make your role decision more firm.

This situation is illustrated by the following case. A young woman in her early twenties visited the dental office for her yearly exam and preventive prophylaxis. During the initial oral examination, the hygienist noted a perio condition on the mandibular anterior facial teeth. The chart from the patient's previous visits did not indicate any similar gingival condition or precautionary measures taken. Handing the patient a hand mirror, the dental hygienist explained the gingival tissue condition on the lower anterior teeth, noting the degree of clefting present, and asked the patient to examine this herself with the mirror. The hygienist suggested the possibility of surgical treatment by a periodontist and explained the need for more thorough daily home dental care by the patient herself. Discussing tooth-brushing habits with the patient, the hygienist learned that the patient brushed once a day, in the morning, with toothpaste. The dental hygienist then suggested that the woman try brushing in the evening, too, this time just with plain water. "I don't have time!" exclaimed the patient, "I don't even have time to watch the ten o'clock news with all the things I have to do, so don't even suggest it!" The hygienist accepted this but informed the patient that without proper daily care, the perio condition would lead to further complications. "Fine," said the young woman, "but I'm not going to brush differently than I do now. I don't have time!"

In this example, the hygienist's role was that of concerned dental professional who not only performed a competent examination but also tried to instruct and educate her patient. The patient responded negatively to the suggestions. If you were the hygienist, what effect would this feedback have on your future recommendations? Holding firmly to your beliefs in preventive dental care, you could try a different persuasive tactic. Or, you could ignore the patient's excuses and do the same thing again. In such situations, you will need to make *some* decision. Most likely your future role behavior will be based on patient feedback.

Patient feedback is determined by patient perceptions of the dental auxiliary and how the patient decodes or interprets the auxiliary's communication. These will vary with each patient. We have not found any helpful studies of how the public views dental auxiliaries. Our own research gives results of a study done in 1980. Attitudes toward "receiving dental care" and attitudes toward "dental hygienists and certified dental assistants" are shown in Figures 4–1 and 4–2.

COMMUNICATION EXERCISE 4–2

List the perceptions the *patient* might have about a *dental hygienist.* In doing this, describe specific behavior and attitudes that fit the perceived role.

List the perceptions a *dental hygienist* might have about the role behavior of *patients.* Be specific in describing attitudes, communication patterns, and behavior.

List the perceptions a patient might have toward a *dental assistant.* Be specific in describing observable behavior that might fit role expectations.

List perceptions a *dental assistant* might have about a *patient.* State specific, observable behavior and kinds of communication.

In the above role descriptions, what differences and similarities do you see in the ways people with different roles see the other?

A number of studies exist on attitudes toward dentists and the reasons patients seek dental care. For example, in a study by the National Opinion Research Center in 1959, 52 percent of the respondents cited money reasons for not seeking dental care, while the second highest category, at 24 percent,

CHARACTERISTIC	ALWAYS %	OCCASIONALLY %	NEVER %
Impersonal	10	51	39
Nasty	0	16	84
Caring	50	48	2
Incompetent	0	27	73
Disinterested	2	54	44
Gentle	43	49	8
Friendly	48	50	2
Careless	0	34	66
Competent	59	41	0
Thorough	64	36	0
Polite	65	33	2
Skilled	64	36	0
Rough	8	47	45
Nervous	2	35	63
Nice	62	38	0
Patient	52	46	2
Humorous	18	68	14
Relaxed	47	49	4
Serious	32	68	0
Sarcastic	0	20	80
Kind	48	52	0

Figure 4–1. Results of survey: Patient perceptions of auxiliary.

From your experience, how do dental assistants and dental hygienists act during dental appointments? Check the most appropriate statement for each characteristic.

How do you feel when you go to a dental office for an appointment? Check the most appropriate statement for each attitude.

ATTITUDE	ALWAYS %	OCCASIONALLY %	NEVER %
Respected	68	30	2
Good	38	40	22
Confident	31	53	16
Uneasy	39	49	12
Anxious	39	49	12
Excited	29	31	40
Nervous	40	50	10
Interested	68	28	4
Scared/Fearful	29	31	40
Hurried	4	55	51
Patient	34	48	18
Appreciated	45	39	16

Figure 4–2. Results of survey: Patient perceptions of dental offices.

cited fear of pain.[2] Contrasting views were found in a study done at Western Washington University which showed that more than half of those who have a "high fear" of dental treatment do not cite pain as a factor in their anxiety over dentistry. Rather, they referred to personal and professional characteristics of the dentists themselves, using such terms as "impersonal," "nasty," "uncaring," "incompetent," "disinterested," "cold," "careless," "rough," "nervous," and "mean."[3] Interestingly, Dr. Arlen D. Lackey, D.D.S., stated during the Kansas Dental Assistants Association meeting in 1980 that the order of public confidence for professional individuals was that bankers were first, dentists second, and physicians third. Patient attitudes and perceptions of this nature, when received by the auxiliary through feedback, could condition the actual role behavior of the auxiliary.

The Dental Context

The fourth influence on your role is the *context* in which you work with patients. Both the physical and the psychological context of a dental setting affect the role. Just as being in a football stadium, a church, a classroom, or a courtroom involves one form of behavior or another, so being in a dental operatory has an influence on role behavior. It is a place where there is some degree of predictable behavior. In some instances, behavior is so predictable that it is a ritual. This is due in part to role expectations (psychological context) and the room's furniture, equipment, and instruments (physical context). How the auxiliary feels about his or her role may be affected also by the wearing of a uniform, having a certificate framed on the wall, wearing a name tag with such initials as RDH or CDA after the name, and so forth. These visible symbols exist to enhance a role. They give the auxiliary credibility. The context itself may give an auxiliary a sense of high self-esteem, competency, and authority. Outside the dental context, in another social setting, the context may influence different role behavior. For example, in the operatory, wearing a white uniform, and sitting on a stool higher than the semiprone patient, a hygienist might speak with certainty and in a confident tone of voice. At a party the same night, the same person might speak with less confidence about a political matter in which others seem to be more knowledgeable.

Context affects role behavior in another way. Berger and Calabrese note that "the basal level of uncertainty a person has about a stranger can be modulated by the communication situation itself."[4] In a dental situation, because much of the activity is predictable on the part of a dental auxiliary, uncertainty may not be as large a factor as it would be in a strange and less structured social situation. On the other hand, there *is* a high degree of uncertainty on the part of patients because even though the physical context may not be strange, the results of a preventive dental checkup are usually unknown in advance. In fact, many patients express anxiety about visiting dental offices simply because they do not know what the results will be after the examination. But it is the *context*—physical and psychological—which creates the anxiety. Away from it, the anxiety decreases (unless there is continuing pain). Another observation by Berger and Calabrese is that "in situations where uncertainty levels are reduced by the situation itself, conversations are likely to begin by focusing on content areas related to the situation."[5] In other words, for a dental auxiliary, talking with the patient about being in the dental context would likely help to diminish uncertainty on the part of the patient.

Because an auxiliary in uniform is a visible part of the context, the context plays a part in the dental auxiliary's role development—both in the eyes of the auxiliary and in the eyes of the patient. Outside this context the roles may be very different. Inside, context provides a common topic of conversation and focuses communication on the subject at hand.

Having considered the importance of your roles, you may wonder what choices you have in your own daily communication. The next chapter will help you examine choices which you might make that are appropriate to your own circumstances.

SUMMARY

This chapter has dealt with roles of dental auxiliaries and of patients. Your role as auxiliary is the identity you have that is related to your particular tasks or responsibilities. In a dental environment, it is seen in the various interpersonal and technical functions you perform on the dental team and with patients. One's perception of self and others helps to define one's role. Thus, your perception of yourself and of your professional identity, as well as your perception of the patient and other members of the dental team, will influence your role behavior. The cultural and social norms of the place in which you work will influence not only your choice of role expectations but also the expectations others have of your role. Roles usually carry emotional involvement, and to be asked to deviate from your role can bring about a defensive reaction. Four situations generally influence the roles of dental auxiliaries: Those in which roles are (1) assigned or (2) chosen, and those in which roles are directly affected by (3) patient feedback and (4) the dental context.

Being aware of the importance your role choice has on your interaction with others will help you analyze and evaluate your communication style so that it is consistent with your role. Such consistent behavior will help others understand who you are in relation to them and how best to communicate with you.

CHAPTER ACTIVITIES

1. From your experience, list as many types of activities as you can recall which match the assigned role of your profession (dental hygienist or dental assistant).
2. In a brief paragraph, write a description of yourself as a dental auxiliary, keeping in mind how you choose to behave in this role. Use lots of descriptive words to be as illustrative as possible. When you are finished, compare your description with that of a classmate or associate to see how that person is similar and how he or she is different.
3. State how perceptions by patients may affect your role related to feedback you might receive from them.
4. Think of physical aspects of a dental context which might influence your role—i.e., how you behave as a dental auxiliary.

REFERENCES

1. Paul Watzlawick, Janet Helmick Beavin, and Don D. Jackson, *Pragmatics of Human Communication* (New York: W. W. Norton & Co. Inc., 1967), p. 31.
2. Peter C. Goulding, "What the Public Thinks of the Dentist and Dental Health," *Journal of the American Dental Association*, 70 (1965), 1211–15. Copyright by the American Dental Association. Reprinted by permission.
3. Joel Greenberg, "Why I Hate the Dentist," *Science News*, 112 (1977), 170. Reprinted with permission from SCIENCE NEWS, the weekly news magazine of science, copyright 1977 by Science Service, Inc.
4. Charles R. Berger and Richard J. Calabrese, "Some Explorations in Initial Interac-

tion and Beyond: Toward a Developmental Theory of Interpersonal Communication," *Human Communication Research*, I, no. 2 (1975), 99–112. Published by permission of Transaction, Inc. from HUMAN COMMUNICATION RESEARCH, Vol. 1, No. 2. Copyright © by the International Communication Association.

5. Ibid.

Communication
Choices

5

When the word "communication" is used in daily conversation, it often is used as a synonym for "speech." But as the two words imply, communication is more than speech. Still, speech is a very important means of communication. Some argue that it is speech that makes human beings unique among the creatures of the earth. Certainly, the importance of speech cannot be ignored. As the late philosopher-theologian Martin Buber said, "The importance of the spoken word . . . is grounded in the fact that it does not want to remain with the speaker. It reaches out toward a hearer, it lays hold of him, it even makes the hearer into a speaker, if perhaps only a silent one."[1] This chapter deals with the communication choices a dental auxiliary can make in the dental context. It deals with speaking in the sense that Buber implies—namely, the speaking with sounds and words, as well as the speaking in ways that are silent.

As you recall from Part I, a *sender encodes* a message which then must be *decoded* by a *receiver*. In Chapters 3 and 4 we explained the importance of perceptions and roles, on the part of both the dental auxiliary and the patient. These are attributes and functions of the sender and receiver. Now we deal more specifically with the encoding and decoding aspects of communication in the delivery of preventive dental care. As we examine these aspects, keep in mind that perceptions and roles play a very important part in determining the encoding and decoding choices which both you and the patient make.

In this chapter we will discuss three types of communication choices: (1) verbal, (2) vocal, and (3) nonverbal–nonvocal. For some readers, this may serve only as a review of material covered more thoroughly in basic college textbooks on speech and communication. We do not intend to try to do in one chapter what an entire textbook can do. What we intend to do is to narrow the topic to aspects which we observe to be most important in the delivery of dental health care.

PERSONAL ASPECTS OF COMMUNICATION

Before discussing each of the three types of communication mentioned above, a preliminary statement needs to be made about three very crucial elements in communication. From the times of ancient Greek and Roman orators, those who have studied communication effectiveness have realized that three elements of human message sending are (1) trust, (2) emotion, and (3) reason.

TRUST.   Trust, which the philosopher Aristotle called *ethos*, is perhaps one of the most crucial aspects of communication between any two or more creatures in the animal world.[2] Between human beings, trust is certainly a key to allowing two people to be open to each other's messages.[3] The old joke that asks, "Would you buy a used car from that man?" is as concise an illustration of this as might be found. It involves the credibility and ethical responsibility which one person has that allows another to believe what he or she says. When delivering preventive dental care, a professional's trustworthiness and credibility allow him or her to be respected, listened to, and believed. If a dental auxiliary, for example, recommends treatment which the patient later discovers was not necessary and may have been recommended only for the sake of making more money for a dentist, credibility will be destroyed and suspicion will be fostered. The ethics of a dental auxiliary affect her communication choices and thus become important to the practice of preventive dentistry.

EMOTION.   This is a human trait which sets the mood, places emphasis, and reinforces the value of message content. Ancient Greeks called this *pathos*. Emotion includes all the human feelings expressed in communication, from happiness and joy to sorrow and disappointment. In a dental setting, the array of emotions may run from the calmness of the dental professional to the anxiety and fear of pain on the part of the patient.

REASON.   Finally, reason is the logical arrangement of ideas in words and sentences to explain and to persuade. Reason, which Greek philosophers called *logos* or logic, depends specifically on words. It is the enemy of falsehood and superstition. During dental health care, reason can help to dispel misconceptions about various dental practices. For example, a soldier went to an Army dental clinic and asked to have a tooth pulled to relieve pain. A dental assistant explained that it is not necessarily a logical deduction to conclude that just because there is a toothache the only solution is to extract the tooth. "Let me take an X-ray. Possibly a root canal may save the tooth," she explained. In this example, reason, combined with credibility and calm emotion, served to educate a patient who had never known other alternatives. [4]

With these three elements—trust, emotion, and reason—in mind, we can look at the choices to make about verbal, vocal, and nonverbal–nonvocal communication.

DEFINITIONS.   *Verbal* communication is the use of words to encode a message. It applies both to speaking and to writing. *Vocal* communication applies to the sounds people make by resonating and controlling air forced out through the vocal tract. *Nonverbal–nonvocal* communication applies to all other behavior that is not speech, writing, or vocal sound. In Figure 5-1, examples are given for verbal, vocal, and nonverbal–nonvocal aspects of communication. They should help you to understand that a person has many communication choices. These choices can include any number of combina-

Figure 5-1. Verbal, vocal, and nonvocal–nonverbal communication.

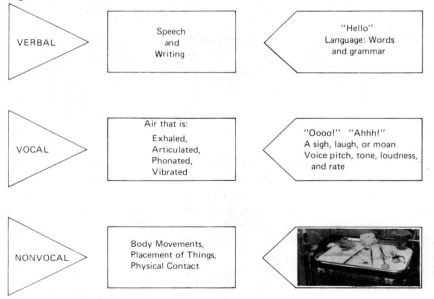

VERBAL	Speech and Writing	"Hello" Language: Words and grammar
VOCAL	Air that is: Exhaled, Articulated, Phonated, Vibrated	"Oooo!" "Ahhh!" A sigh, laugh, or moan Voice pitch, tone, loudness, and rate
NONVOCAL	Body Movements, Placement of Things, Physical Contact	

tions of verbal, vocal, and nonverbal–nonvocal behavior. The remainder of this chapter is a brief survey of these choices.

Looking at the chart, you can see that there is more to making communication choices than simply selecting words. In fact, patients receiving preventive dental care have little chance to use speech because of the semifixed position of their mouths and their inability to use their articulators (tongue, teeth, and lips) in normal fashion. But keep in mind that you do have choices about your communication. The following diagram (Figure 5–2), illustrating the speech chain, helps to show not only how speech is processed but also that speech—and all intentional communication—begins in the brain. [5]

VERBAL COMMUNICATION

Words are simply symbols of our thoughts. They are a code. Hence, using words in speaking and writing is a way of encoding a message. In this section, verbal communication is examined under the subheadings of (1) meaning, (2) style, and (3) appropriateness.

Meaning

Basically, words can have *connotative* meaning and *denotative* meaning. Connotative meaning is the meaning implied, while denotative meaning is the literal or "dictionary" meaning of a word. Science and the legal profession attempt to deal strictly in denotative meanings, being as precise as possible. In so doing, very technical and academic-sounding words emerge. Conversational talk often includes more connotative than denotative meanings in words. The difference is seen in this example:

"She's a dog"—*denotes* a canine animal.

"She's a dog"—*connotes* an unattractive female human being.

Students of general semantics believe that words by themselves do not have meanings, but rather that meanings are found in how other persons perceive the meaning. So, they say, there can never really be an accurately worded statement which would completely describe anything in all cases for all people.

Slang often falls under the category of connotative language because of the use of one word in one speech community may mean the opposite for another group of people. For example, "bad" could mean "good" and a "bad mother" could mean "tough man," depending on the context.

A caution then, is to never assume that your patient understands the same meaning of the word that you intend, no matter how simple it may seem

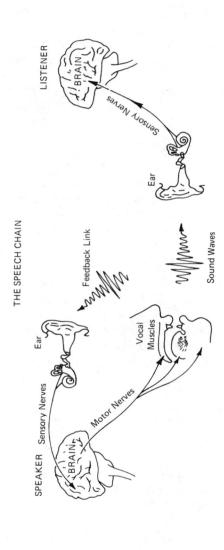

Figure 5–2. The speech chain. (Figure 5–8 from *The Speech Chain* by Peter B. Denes and Elliot N. Pinson. Copyright © 1963 by Bell Telephone Laboratories, Inc. Reprinted by permission of Doubleday & Company, Inc.)

to be to you. Also, be aware that although it is more accurate to use words that are technically correct to describe the dental structures of the oral cavity, your patient may not have those words in his or her vocabulary.[6]

Style

Words are selected from an individual's own vocabulary and arranged in particular ways, using grammar and syntax, to form sentences and verbal expressions. The way this is done is referred to as *style*. Here are two examples of the same idea encoded in two different styles:

> "My God! You haven't been brushing or flossing!"
> "Your teeth have no cavities, but it looks like we'll need to spend some time removing a large buildup of calculus and stain."

Style often carries connotative meaning, just as does a word. In the above examples, the first style takes on an implication of shock and value judgment. It could be a condemnation which the listener could perceive in a very defensive way, creating an unwillingness to openly discuss preventive dental treatment. The second statement is less judgmental and includes a positive comment ("no cavities") which likely would make the patient feel that the speaker is a likeable, caring person. The statement about the condition of the teeth is an objective, matter-of-fact description, intending neither shock nor judgment.

Your own reasons for communicating will influence your style. From the example given above, we can arrive at five reasons to use language which govern the choice of style. These are:

1. To describe
2. To inform, make known
3. To instruct, educate, teach a skill
4. To manage or alter behavior, persuade, motivate
5. To evaluate, judge, give praise or blame

Following are examples of each of these reasons as they affect stylistic choice:

1. *Description*	"*There is* heavy calculus on the outside of your upper back teeth."
2. *Information*	"Calculus *is what makes* the tissues around your teeth red and inflamed."
3. *Instruction*	"Here is *how to* brush and floss in order to prevent further buildup of calculus."
4. *Behavior management*	"You have done a very *good* job of caring *for these teeth and gums in the front*

(positive reinforcement); doing this well on the area in the back should *result* in healthy gums and teeth that have no calculus at all" *(desired behavior)*.

5. *Evaluation*   "This is a *good* job here! You *should* do it this same way in all areas of your mouth."

ACCURACY. In any health-care situation, specific statements describe specific illnesses, parts of the anatomy, behavior, and so forth. The context of health care itself narrows the focus of the subject matter. This, in turn, narrows the communication choices, which, in turn, narrow the limits of language. To be accurate is to state specifically what is intended. Of course, as stated earlier in this chapter, connotative meanings and denotative meanings can garble the intended meaning in verbal communication. Nevertheless, it is helpful to a listener if the speaker is specific and concrete, rather than general and vague.

General statements may or may not apply to the specific individual you are addressing. For example,

"Sometimes people with a similar condition have little or no problems at all; sometimes a surgical procedure is required."

The patient is left wondering if *he* is one of the "people" and if *this* time is one of the "sometimes." And what does "similar condition" mean? Does it mean *this* condition, here, in this patient's mouth? And the phrase "little or no" is ambiguous. It would be more specific and concrete to say,

"The condition on this tooth (pointing to a radiograph) is called a periodontal abscess, which the doctor might recommend being lacerated and drained."

Here, acuracy is maintained while still keeping the statement simple.

OBJECTIVE DESCRIPTION. To use description effectively, a dental auxiliary should choose nonjudgmental, objective statements. Such statements use facts, numbers, statistics, and nonornamental words. In contrast, a judgmental statement uses such words as "should," "ought," "good," "bad," and other value-laden words. Descriptive words are best for recording the dental history on patient charts as well as for straightforward statements to a patient about the condition of his or her oral cavity. Nonevaluative description can be used together with simplicity and accuracy, but it may require a conscientious effort for a speaker to do so. A good example is the last statement used in the above section under accuracy.

Judgmental statements include:

"You should have come here six months ago."
"You do a great job!"
"The condition of this patient's gums is bad." (to a dentist)

Nonjudgmental and objective alternatives are:

"A regular six-month checkup allows us to catch these problems in their early stages when they are easily treated without serious complications."
"The way you brush and floss at home has been effective in keeping your teeth and gums healthy."
"This patient's teeth have occlusal weak facets."

Factual description relies upon details, accurate dental terminology, specific dates, names, and numbers.

ILLUSTRATION.   Illustration as used here refers to wording a message in a manner that provides a mental image for the listener. *Adverbs* and *adjectives* help to describe and more clearly illustrate something. *Analogies* also help to illustrate a situation by comparing something in a known category with something in an unknown category to help the listener understand the unknown. *Contrast* also helps by illustrating how one thing is unlike another.
     Here are some examples of illustration:

"Mrs. Jones, do you remember ever having a sliver in your finger? The area around the sliver was sore, red, and puffy. The same thing is happening in your mouth. See this calculus? As it builds up on your teeth, the tissues around it get rubbed raw, just like around the sliver. They're red, puffy, and bleed spontaneously when I touch them."

In this example, the analogy compares something the patient knows from past experience with something the speaker is trying to explain. This is an analogy. The example also uses descriptive adjectives (sore, red, puffy) to help illustrate the condition clearly for the patient.
     To illustrate something, it is useful to use words with which the listener is familiar. When using analogies it is only helpful when you compare things that are unknown (i.e., what you are trying to explain) with things that are *familiar* to the listener. You will need to know the person's background and general vocabulary before assuming that your illustrative technique is effective. Analogies are often most helpful with persons who have no previous experience in dental care as well as people who have impaired vision and cannot see what you are doing.

What Is Appropriate?

In a dental environment, there are three basic types of talk: "small talk," which helps you introduce yourself to the patient and can help to put the patient at ease; "dental talk," which includes the biographical and dental information obtained in an interview, as well as the more technical and care-oriented talk that goes on in the operatory, relating directly to personalized preventive dental care; and "business talk," which generally deals with appointments and financial matters. Each kind of talk has appropriate words. As a general rule, the words you use should fit *you*, the professional *setting*, and the *other person*. Using your own generational, ethnic, racial, or regional slang which is appropriate to you outside the dental environment probably is not appropriate in the dental office. On the other hand, using very formal and "professional-sounding" talk which is uncomfortable to you and which seems phony to you probably will sound that way to the patient. The setting, however, is a professional one and not a social one; language suitable to the delivery of preventive dental care, and to you as a person well-educated in this field, is what is appropriate.

Being aware of feedback from the other person will help you know if your language is suitable to that person. The patient's age, amount of formal education, type of work, regional and ethnic background (even if he or she no longer lives and associates with persons from that background), religious identity, and prior experience in dental offices and clinics are all helpful kinds of biographical data that can assist you in making appropriate verbal choices when you are talking with that person. If you work with young children or with persons who have communication difficulties (impaired speech, hearing, and/or sight), there may be another person in the room with the patient for assistance and observation. Some of these special concerns will be discussed in a later chapter; however, in such cases keep both persons in mind so that you use a vocabulary both can understand. You need not talk "kiddie talk" with children; but you do need to be aware of the extent of their vocabulary and, for younger children, try to keep multisyllabic words to a minimum.

These are only general guidelines. If you keep the stylistic suggestions in mind which are included in this section and be aware of what is suitable to *you*, the *setting*, and the *other person*, then chances are that your verbal communication will be appropriate in your work as a dental auxiliary.

VOCAL COMMUNICATION

Vocal communication can be defined as the use of sounds produced in the vocal tract to transmit a message and set the mood for verbal communication in speech. This section should help you understand that vocal communication can be either used by itself without words, or used in speech *with* words. A giggle, a sigh, and a moan are vocal but nonverbal; each sends a message. Likewise, the meaning of words spoken with a high-pitched sound can be altered to mean something else with a low-pitched sound. Thus, vocal communication can be either verbal or nonverbal and thereby be useful in conveying the message as you intend it to be understood.

Sound Production

Sound begins when the *diaphragm* forces *air* out from the *lungs*, through the *trachea*, through the *vocal folds* in the *larynx* where the air begins to *vibrate*, on through the *pharynx*, and into the *oral* and *nasal cavities* where the vibrating air is *resonated*, then over the *tongue*, *teeth*, and *lips*, where it is shaped and articulated. Until it reaches the articulators, it is vocal and not verbal.

In human sound production, breathing, tonal quality, amplitude (loudness), and pitch are the key elements affecting vocal communication. These elements used by themselves (nonverbally) or with articulated speech assist us in communicating meaning and emotion. A loud "Ahhh!" may imply pain, while a softly voiced "Ahhh!" may mean relief from pain. Moaning, sighing, giggling, and other vocal sounds have different connotations depending on the emphasis and variety used to produce the sounds. Emphasis is accomplished by a rising or falling pitch, and by increased or decreased loudness.

Words also can be given connotative meanings by means of changes in volume and pitch. You can experience this yourself by increasing either the pitch or the volume on the italicized words in the following sentences. As you do this, imagine the connotation perceived by a patient in this hypothetical statement by a dental hygienist talking to a dentist:

> "*Look* at the fractured M.O.D. on number 30!"
> "Look at the *fractured* M.O.D. on number 30!"
> "Look at the fractured *M.O.D.* on number 30!"
> "Look at the fractured M.O.D. on number *30*!"

A dental auxiliary needs to realize that not only are words conveying messages; so also is the vocal aspect of speech. The emphasis and variety used assist the communicator in encoding and aid the listener in decoding.

Articulation and Pronunciation

In addition to the vocal aspects of volume, tone, and pitch—which may be used either with or without words—there are two more vocal aspects that generally are associated strictly with speech. These are *articulation* and *pronunciation*. Articulation is the formation of vocal sounds by the tongue, teeth, and lips into specific speech sounds, including the words used in speech. Pronunciation is the manner of articulation that causes the word sounds to be understood in a particular language. Differences in pronunciations of the same words in English in various parts of the United States and, of course, in various parts of the world, make this a difficult topic to discuss in terms of what is "correct." However, it does influence the interpretation of vocal–verbal communication.

Being conscious of your articulation and your pronunciation will allow you to be aware of all the vowels and consonants that should be vocalized in speech. The vowels are

a, e, i, o, u, and sometimes *y* and *w*

These are formed by various shapes of the mouth and lips. Consonants are all the remaining letters of the alphabet. Their pronunciation involves the tongue, teeth, and lips working in various combinations to stop and release the air being used in speech, or to allow the air to be forced through a partially closed or tight passage between the articulators. There are many basic speech textbooks as well as diction manuals that can help you learn more about this aspect of speech production. Your librarian should be able to assist you in locating these for your own individual study.

RATE.   One additional aspect of speech production is *rate.* How rapidly or slowly words are spoken affects the meaning and interpretation of speech. A rapid rate affects other aspects, too, especially articulation and pronunciation. Rapidly rushing through individual words can cause a speaker to drop out sounds from words which should be included. Middle consonant sounds and final consonant sounds are often the victims of very rapid speech. For example, try to say the following sentence at the three speeds recommended and notice how you articulate the sounds in the words:

RATE
Very Slowly

Normal   "I will take this slow-speed handpiece with a little
Conversational   rubber cup with polishing paste to buff your teeth.
Rate   Then the dentist will examine your teeth."
Very Fast

Some common articulation problems with this sentence could be with the following words and phrases:

Word/Phrase	Common Misarticulation
"take this"	"take 'is"
"handpiece"	"han'piece"
"little"	"liddle"
"polishing"	"polishin' "
"to buff"	"t' buff"
"dentist"	"den'ist" or "dendist"

Pronunciation of the final "er" in "rubber" has various regionally acceptable variations which would make the word "rubbuh."

Running sounds together so that it is difficult to distinguish between them, dropping sounds out of words, or adding sounds that are not in the word are common articulation and pronunciation problems.

What Is Appropriate?

Speech is a very individual and often personal activity for each of us. College students often tell us that they dread having to give a speech in front of other people, especially their friends. In many cases, they do not want others to pay that much attention to their speech habits. It is a personal part of their identity which they prefer to have others accept as it is. However, if communication is important to your delivery of preventive dentistry, care must be taken to make the vocal of communication as clearly understood as possible.

The first general rule is (1) *to be aware of the vocal aspects of your own speech*. Use a tape recorder to listen to how others hear you. Also (2) *pay attention to ways in which other people use vocal emphasis and variety in volume, pitch, and tone and what influence this has on how you perceive them*. What helps you as a listener? Does the high-pitched nasal tone bother you and detract from what the speaker is saying? Does a voice with a deeply resonant tone have a different effect than one with a less resonant tone? On radio broadcasts, listen to the types of voices that appeal to you; announcers' voices are a primary consideration for their employment, based on how they appeal to the largest possible audience. Because you must deal with a diversified "audience" as a dental auxiliary, in dental care, a third general rule is (3) *to use general American English pronunciation*. This is what current dictionaries describe phonetically in the pronunciation guides. It is also used by people who must deal with large audiences, those who travel extensively in their jobs, and those who announce news on national television and radio.[7] Regionalisms and slang are generally inappropriate, both in word choice and in pronunciation. Accents may be appropriate in the region in which the accent is common. But because of the mobility of modern society, we recommend that you develop an ability to use general American vocal communication—namely, that which would be easily understood by anyone who understands spoken American English. Careful articulation also will help Americans to be understood more easily by those who speak non–American English, and those who speak English as a second language. This advice does not mean that you give up your individuality or your ability to speak in ways acceptable to your own region or ethnic background. Rather, it means adding to your speech abilities, if necessary, an ability to talk to a broader audience than your friends and family.

There are four types of situations in which dental auxiliaries might find the vocal aspects of communication to be significant in dealing with patients. They begin with (1) telephone conversations, and proceed through (2) casual conversation with a patient as you walk to the operatory and get situated for (3) the interview, and finally through (4) dental-care procedures.

TELEPHONE. On the telephone, vocal communication is more noticeable because of the absence of visual communication. The tone and pitch of a receptionist or dental auxiliary can easily convey attitude and emotion, care or indifference, friendliness or "just plain business." A Certified Dental Assistant told us, while discussing communication topics for this book, that she has heard receptionists' voices sound "so mean" that if she were the patient she would never go to that dentist's office again. Some dental offices do not have a separate receptionist; instead, dental auxiliaries answer the phone and make appointments. Whoever it may be, this is the first person (and, if this person also keeps the books, the last person) a patient talks with concerning the dental appointment. A person's tone of voice contributes to the initial impression that sets the emotional mood for the patient's entire dental appointment. A calm, friendly tone gets the appointment off on a good note.

Articulation is also important, both over the telephone and in person. Make sure that names, dates, times, types of dental procedures done, and other factual information is clearly heard. "Thursday at 10 o'clock" could sound like "Tuesday at 1 o'clock" if a speaker's volume is so low at the beginning of words that all a listener can hear is the "-sday" and the "-n' o'clock" sounds.

CASUAL CONVERSATION. From the welcome in the waiting room to the seating of a patient in the dental chair, casual conversation can be used to put a patient at ease. Tone, pitch, and volume all contribute to setting this mood. A harsh, loud voice might make a patient tense before any dental treatment has even begun. Children, especially, appreciate a kind attitude expressed through the tone of voice of a dental auxiliary.

INTERVIEWS. In an interview, the conversation may take a businesslike tone. You should, of course, speak loudly enough for the patient to hear you. Diction is also important to make it as easy as possible for the patient to understand each word you use in the interview. Mumbling through the material because you have said it so many times before and because you are tired of repeating the same old questions does not help the patient answer the questions. So, instead of having to repeat yourself more often than necessary, speak clearly and distinctly the first time.

DENTAL-CARE PROCEDURES.   During the delivery of dental care, the agitation of the amalgamator or the sound of the high-speed handpiece may interfere with your vocal communication. Increase your volume if necessary; or better, wait until the equipment noise has stopped.

   A brief word needs to be said about persons with impaired sight and hearing. Those with little or no vision rely greatly on vocal inflections to understand the meaning of words in speech. Speech becomes more important as a communication medium. Vocal tone, pitch, and volume, with meaningful variety and emphasis, will assist these patients in understanding clearly what sighted patients can see. Persons with impaired hearing may not need you to shout at them. It may be the pitch or tone of your voice that will assist them to hear you. If they are deaf and read lips, your careful articulation (with tongue, teeth, and lips) will make it easy for them to "see" your words being formed.

   Being aware of feedback from the patient will help you adjust to the situation, as in every other communication situation. Becoming acquainted with persons of all ages with sight and hearing impairments will help you know what is appropriate and what is not.

   Thus far, we have dealt with verbal and vocal aspects of communication, those usually associated with speech. There is more to communication than words and sounds. As we explained in Part I, we use all the senses to receive messages and many types of nonvocal and nonverbal behavior to send messages. This, then, is the final aspect of the personal communication choices discussed in this chapter: nonverbal–nonvocal communication.

NONVERBAL–NONVOCAL COMMUNICATION

At the beginning of this chapter we quoted Martin Buber's observation that a "speaker" can be silent. Deaf persons and those who learn to be interpreters for them are probably more conscious than are hearing persons of the many nonverbal–nonvocal ways in which we can communicate without speech. In this final section on communication choices, we discuss nonverbal–nonvocal communication as it applies to the delivery of dental health care. Because it is popular to refer to this simply as "nonverbal" communication, this is the word we use during the remainder of this chapter. However, it should be kept in mind that we are also referring to nonvocal communication as well in this last section.

In the communication model for dental auxiliaries we listed the five senses and gave corresponding encoders for each. With the exception of the sense of hearing, all the rest may be considered as nonverbal communication elements. Therefore, here we shall elaborate on these as they apply to you. The following are eight distinct ways in which people communicate:

1. Body movements and facial expressions
2. Distance or proximity between two or more people
3. Touch
4. Object placement and environmental organization
5. Odor
6. Status
7. Time usage and value
8. Dress and grooming

There are many other ways which anthropologists and communication researchers identify as nonverbal means of communication.[8] These eight, we believe, relate most closely to your work as a dental auxiliary. As you study this section, keep in mind that being aware of your own nonverbal behavior is as important as being aware of your patient's nonverbal behavior. In interpersonal communication, both (or all) people send nonverbal messages, because practically everything we do has message value.

Body Movements and Facial Expressions

In the process of preventive dental care, body movements and facial expressions are very obvious to those in the operatory. Because of the patient's relative immobility and restricted head movement, what you say with hand gestures and, especially, facial expressions, may be as important as what you say with words. The following photographs show a variety of facial expressions and hand movements which may say a variety of things, depending on the verbal communication that accompanies them.

You, as a dental auxiliary, will be able to notice various facial expressions and bodily movements on the part of your patient. The patient, with dental work being done, has a difficult time using speech. Tightly gripping an armrest, squirming, flinching, blinking at a bright light, and nervously wiggling feet are nonverbal body movements you may notice.

Just as you observe these messages coming from your patient, the patient is likewise observing you. Many nonverbal messages are sent by choice. Your smile, your frown, or your somber face may be perceived as a message and your patient perception will contribute to the patient's subse-

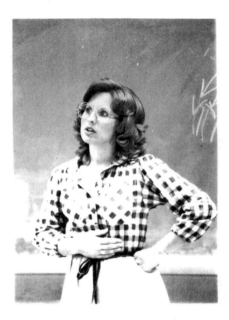

Figure 5-3. Nonverbal messages clarify verbal communication. Notice, in Figures 5-3 through 5-7, the specific hand and arm movements and facial expressions that communicate meaning.

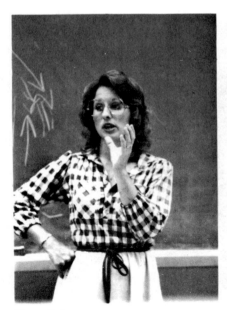

Figure 5-4.

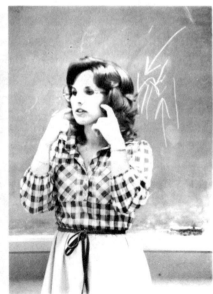

Figure 5-5.

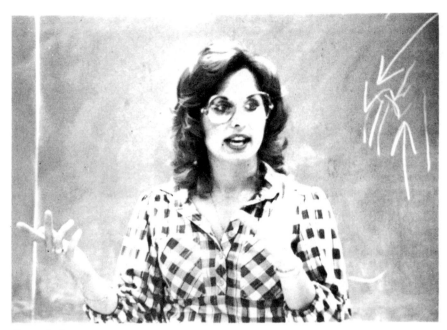

Figure 5-6.

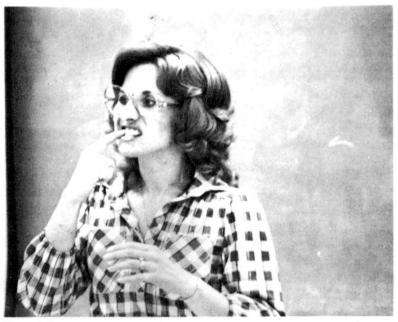

Figure 5-7.

quent behavior. If you have direct eye contact with a patient, this may tell the other person that you are interested in him or her, and that you are listening. Infrequent eye contact could indicate disinterest. A smile while working with an apprehensive patient may help to calm and relax the individual. Careful, precise hand movements when laying out dental instruments on a tray in front of a patient may be a nonverbal message that you are a careful and precise person, knowledgeable about your work and not apt to fumble and bumble during dental treatment.

Distance

How close you are in relation to others in the operatory constitutes another nonverbal message. Proximity is a form of message. At a formal dinner party, where one guest sits in relation to other guests is often determined by the relative "social importance" of each guest. In a dental setting, dental professionals and a patient, by necessity, must be close during dental procedures. However, proximity is still a factor to be aware of in your communication choices. For example, how close are you when interviewing a patient? And where do you place yourself in the room in relation to the patient's direct line of sight? If you are behind a patient, the headrest restricts the patient's head from turning to look at you when you are talking or working. This might con-

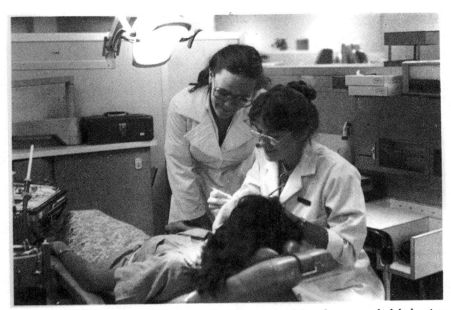

Figure 5–8. Patient perceptions are often determined by the nonverbal behavior displayed on the part of the dental auxiliary. A smile and good eye contact tell the patient you are interested in him or her.

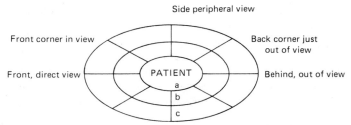

Figure 5-9. Proximity diagram. Viewing the operatory from above, the patient is in a semireclining position in the center of imaginary concentric circles. Your position and your distance from the patient could fit any of the segments within this diagram. The width of each circle is about 12 inches. The best position for dental procedures is in circle a. In circle b, the suitable position for interviewing would be near the front corner and in view of the patient. Circles a, b, and c indicate the general vicinity in which CDAs assist during most routine dental procedures.

vey the message that you are doing something secretive which the patient should not see. This could heighten anxiety. Or it may tell the patient that, by avoiding face-to-face eye contact, you do not want to get to know the patient very well. If you are out of sight, the patient could feel alone. And whether you stand or sit at eye level with the patient, you may seem to be more sympathetic and likeable than if you stood or sat a foot or more higher than the patient. When you literally look down on a patient, the patient may figuratively feel "put down." Being on the same level as another person has both physical and psychological implications, carrying both denotative and connotative messages. In Figure 5-9 you can see how distance and proximity can be evaluated for your own nonverbal behavior in relation to a patient, who sits in the center of the circles.

An interesting relationship between proximity and familiarity with a particular room has been noticed in a study by J. J. Edney. The results of this study indicated that both past experience and expectation of future experience with a room leads to a closer interpersonal distance. This is one of the few studies of nonverbal communication with direct application to the unique context of a dental operatory. It would indicate that close proximity is expected by patient and dental professionals because of the nature of the operatory itself.[9] Figures 5-10a and 5-10b show examples of typical operatory situations involving a patient with members of the dental team and their relative distances.

Touch

In many instances, touching is an intimate form of communication. When parents hold and hug a child, this carries a strong message of closeness, love, and security for the child. The value of a human touch apparently does not

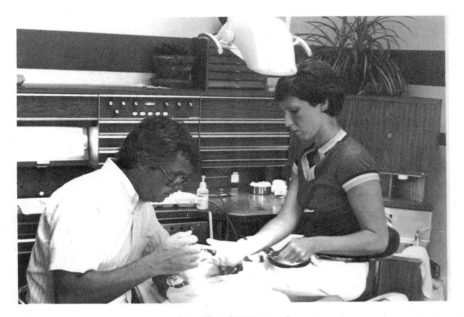

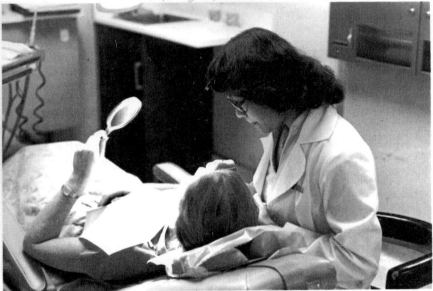

Figure 5–10 (a and b). Examples of typical operatory situations showing proximity of the patient and dental professionals.

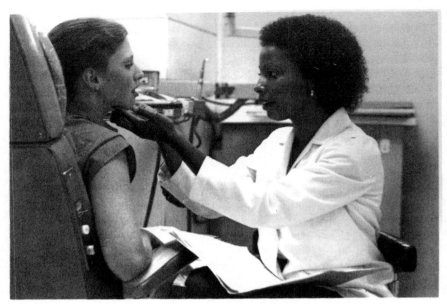

Figure 5-11. A gentle touch by a dental auxiliary during oral examinations communicates a caring attitude and generates a feeling of trust in the patient.

diminish as long as we live. In the practice of preventive dental care, there is constant touching by the dental professional—placing the dental napkin on a patient, palpating a patient's tongue, holding an upper lip, and so forth. Because of this the patient again receives messages about how the professional cares about both the work and the patient. Rough, jerking hand movements on a patient's jaw may send a message of indifference, resulting in patient reactions of noncooperative behavior. Accidental touching, such as swinging an elbow into a patient, backing into a patient, and other unnecessary bumping carries a negative message value.

Objects

Most dental facilities have a sterile, businesslike appearance. Consequently, what a patient *sees* (or *feels*, in the case of sight-impaired persons) tells him or her something about the work being done in the room. All the objects in the room—such as instruments, mechanical equipment, pictures on walls, diplomas, and so forth—as well as their color and condition, have message value and should not be ignored. You can imagine the impression given by the patched dental chair or the broken cable cover in Figures 5-12 and 5-13. Careful attention to general repair and orderliness is important.

One dental hygienist working in a pedodontic office places a collection

Figure 5-12. If you were a patient, what messages about the delivery of dental care would you have from the scenes pictured here and in Figure 5-13? The physical environment of the dental office carries an important message to the patient.

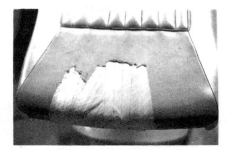

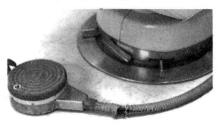

Figure 5-13.

of drawings done by her young patients on one wall. These are at the eye level of children sitting in the dental chair. Above these, she also has two colorful charts illustrating kinds of foods that are good for healthy teeth and some that are harmful. In addition, at eye level of the parents as they enter the room with their children, is the hygienist's certificate, stating that she is a Registered Dental Hygienist in that state. The wall colors in her operatory are soft, pastel blue, which gives a peaceful effect. These objects, together with the regular dental equipment, help to create an environment in which the young patients learn to feel comfortable. With careful planning, a dental office itself can "say" just what the dental auxiliary wants to say.

Odor

Apart from the cultural values of cleanliness which mass-media advertisers constantly try to teach us, the odors that accompany dental care are important factors in the interpersonal communication of the patient and dental auxiliary. General cleanliness in the operatory, including the smell of the air, may send a quick message to a patient that "here is an operatory that is O.K. to be in for treatment." A stuffy room with strong odors of any kind could give an immediate nonverbal message that "this is an uncomfortable place to be." Aside from the general atmosphere in the operatory, odors from dental chemicals such as Lysol spray and zinc-oxide-eugenol, can say to a patient, "Yes, this is definitely a dental operatory." People with vision impairments may notice odors more distinctly. Those entering a dental operatory for the first time may find that different odors cause momentary uneasiness which may contribute to an already-existing sense of anxiety.

Your own personal cleanliness—the use of mouthwash, soap, deodorant, and fresh clothing each day—also carry message value. How clean you smell to others may give you high credibility as a competent dental professional. Further, the general socially acceptable attributes of interpersonal behavior includes the faint to moderate use of perfumes, colognes, and other aromatics. However, what may be acceptable for a social occasion may not be appropriate in a dental context. Because of the close proximity of the dental auxiliary and patient, this becomes important to total work effectiveness.

Status

Status is a person's rank or position in an identifiable group of people, such as a dental team. As mentioned earlier, the word "patient" itself carries an implied status of one who needs help, one who is unhealthy or one who is passively dependent. In any of these conditions, some patients may tend to see themselves in a lower-status position than those on the dental team, from the receptionist on "up" to the dentist. In fact, dental office and clinic staffs may be perceived in terms of a hierarchical status structure (see Part IV) by the patient, as well as by staff members themselves. While status does not relate to the senses directly (although sight plays a principal function here), the "five E's" mentioned earlier come into play here more, and thus feelings about status are part of the total nonverbal–nonvocal communication picture.

In interviews conducted for this textbook, the authors discovered a communication trend based on status. Although further samples would be needed to determine how universal these trends are among patients and dental staff members, the following have emerged which illustrate the point:

1. Patients tend to feel more free to talk openly with dental auxiliaries about their anxieties and complaints about the dentist, and personal problems, than they do with dentists.
2. Patients tend to feel more free to talk openly with CDAs about their lack of knowledge about specific dental procedures than they do with RDHs or dentists.
3. Patients tend to feel more free to talk with dental auxiliaries than with dentists about financial problems that may hinder them from seeking recommended treatment.
4. Patients perceive the highest status as belonging to the dentist. Registered Dental Hygienists, Certified Dental Assistants, noncertified dental assistants, office managers, and receptionists follow in this relative order.

We could postulate that status, perceived by the patient in the order just cited, would account for the degree of communication with different staff members. To carry this hypothesis further, the person of highest status would be the one most distant in status from the patient, as long as they are in the dental context; the more distant, the more difficult to talk with. If your observations are similar to ours, you can pay attention to the communication content and general attitude a patient has with you in comparison with other staff members. If there is a noticeable difference, then status reinforced by labels ("doctor," "hygienist," "assistant," etc.) likely has an influence on nonverbal communication. Understanding role behavior, as described in Chapter IV, will help you understand more about the influence of status in communication.

Time

Time, as a form of nonverbal communication, refers to the message value of how time is used. This, according to Edward T. Hall, is a culturally determined message.[10] Different cultures have different perceptions of time. In North America, for example, being "on time" for an appointment means more than simply arriving punctually at the predetermined time. There is also an implicit message in being "on time"—namely, that it is a virtue to be punctual. To arrive 30 minutes or more after an appointment is considered more than just being "late." It can carry such implicit messages as "lack of consideration," "disorganization," "inefficiency," and "rudeness." A patient late for an appointment might also be saying, by the delay, that he or she is afraid of what might happen at the dental office.

Your use of time as a dental auxiliary is of equal importance. Patients who put a high value on being on time, or who use the motto "time is money," are apt to resent waiting more than 15 minutes in a waiting room. Likewise, they are likely to resent sitting alone in a dental operatory waiting for dental care to begin. Maintaining a realistic appointment schedule sends a nonverbal message to patients that you respect their time, realize the value of their time, and are yourself an organized and efficient professional. These are values common in general American and European cultures. Time does not carry the same message value in all cultures, or in all subcultures within the American society. You should be conscious of this cultural aspect of nonverbal communication when working with patients from ethnic and national backgrounds different from your own.

Dress and Grooming

Dress and personal appearance have long been ways in which people in all cultures have told others about themselves. Often, dress reflects status and self-image. Many corporations have dress and grooming codes for employees, believing that the public may judge the company's efficiency and responsibility via nonverbal messages related to personal appearance.

Special dress, such as uniforms worn in a dental office, helps everyone identify the role each person plays. In a hospital or large dental clinic, uniforms take on even more importance than in a small dental office. Consider Figures 5–14, 5–15, and 5–16. In Figure 5–14, the CDA is wearing a traditional white cap and a colorful plaid uniform, distinguishing her from a student dentist in a university dental school clinic. Both wear white jackets. In Figure 5–15, the CDA wears a colorful uniform, designating her position, while the RDH wears a traditional white jacket. Figure 5–16 shows a male dentist in private practice wearing a casual sport shirt and a CDA wearing a contemporary smock suitable for private practice. In this latter situation, patients know the role of each person on the dental team, making clothing distinctions simply a matter of personal preference rather than a matter of symbolic necessity. In a large public clinic, clothing distinctions have more symbolic value to both the patients and those who work there.

General neatness, as opposed to extremes in fashion and grooming, would likely say to a patient that "the business of this dental auxiliary is to care for my teeth, not to impress me with her wardrobe and hairstyle." This would apply either to casual clothing or to uniforms. Social custom is prob-

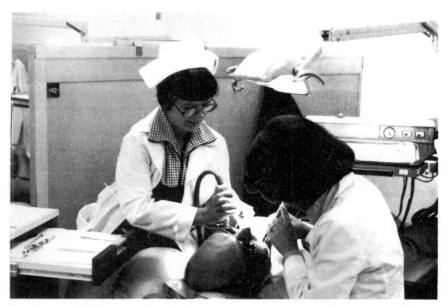

Figure 5–14. Uniforms on dental professionals help identify specific roles for patients. However, in the three photographs in Figures 5–14 through 5–16 there are two dentists. Can you identify them by their dress?

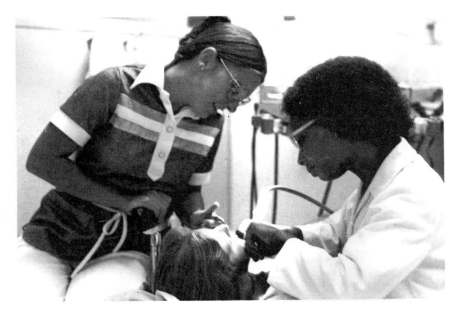

Figure 5-15.

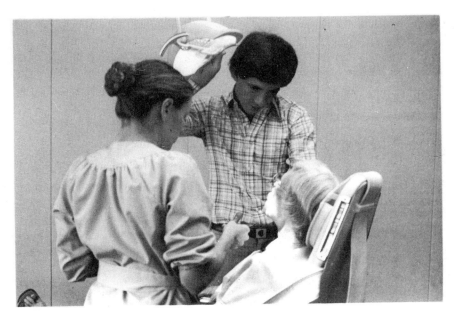

Figure 5-16.

ably the best guide. Yet a common factor in any health-related profession is cleanliness and neatness, for the message value these attributes send is of a disease-free environment and efficient professional behavior. Without elaborating further on this aspect of nonverbal communication, suffice it to say that this is one of the communication choices which dental auxiliaries make each day.

What Is Appropriate?

Nonverbal–nonvocal communication choices, like verbal and vocal choices, must take into account both individual integrity and social acceptability. Individual standards, self-concept, role, and status expectations influence nonverbal choices. Without sacrificing those aspects of your personal behavior which make your personality unique, the choices you make about communication in a dental setting should be appropriate to the social and professional norms in both the community and the specific office or clinic in which you work.

There are three techniques by which you can observe and evaluate your own nonverbal behavior. One way is to use a mirror, watching your own natural behavior as you talk to an imaginary patient. Role playing will help you accomplish a realistic scene. Look for body movements, hand gestures, and facial expressions as you talk. A second technique is to use videotape. Most dental schools, community colleges, and technical institutes have video cameras and recording equipment which you might use individually or as a class. Role playing via videotape is much easier to observe than watching yourself in a mirror. You can evaluate your nonverbal behavior more objectively in this way and replay the tape as often as you wish. A third technique is to observe feedback from others as they respond to your own nonverbal communication. This is the most realistic evaluation of all, although it may be difficult to be objective in your evaluation.

If you monitor your own nonverbal behavior in any of the above three ways, you will be aware of the ways others see you. And, if you are surprised to see that some of your behavior projects a negative feeling, you can make conscientious choices to change or alter the behavior. Just as you can increase your verbal ability and add meaningful variety and emphasis to your vocal delivery, you can make your nonverbal behavior appropriate to your communication goals.

SUMMARY

In this chapter, discussions have centered around the verbal, vocal, and nonverbal communication choices which a dental auxiliary makes in the dental environment. The three elements necessary for effective message sending are trust, emotion, and reason. *Trust* is the key allowing two people to send open messages to one another. *Emotion* sets the mood of the message that is sent. *Reason* is the logical arrangement of the ideas in the message. *Verbal communication* is the use of words to encode a message. It refers to the writing and speaking aspect of communication. *Vocal communication* is the use of sounds produced in the vocal equipment to transmit a message and set the mood for the communication transaction. *Nonverbal–nonvocal communication* refers to all other aspects associated with sending a message which do not involve speech, writing, or vocal sounds.

Verbal communication can be examined in terms of meaning, style, and appropriateness (accuracy) of the message. In vocal communication, the key elements of the discussion to remember are breathing, tonal quality, amplitude (loudness), and pitch. *Articulation* is the formation of vocal sounds by the tongue, teeth, and lips into speech sounds. *Pronunciation* is the manner of articulation that creates sounds that can be understood. Using appropriate speech is important when the dental auxiliary is answering the telephone, talking with patients on a casual basis, talking with patients in the operatory, and during the interviewing process. There are three general guidelines for appropriate communication choices for dental auxiliaries: (1) be aware of the vocal aspect of your own speech; (2) pay attention to ways other people use vocal emphasis and variety in volume, pitch, and tone and what influence this has on how you perceive them; and (3) use general American English pronunciation at all times in the dental environment. We communicate nonverbally as well as nonvocally via body movements and facial expressions; distance or proximity between ourselves and others; touch, objects within the dental office and environmental organization, odor, status, time usage and value, and dress and grooming. Volumes of literature have been written on this subject, thus the discussion was limited here to the most appropriate aspects relating to the dental environment. Three techniques by which individuals can observe and evaluate their own nonverbal behavior are to (1) use a mirror and watch your own natural behaviors as you talk with an imaginary patient; (2) use a videotape and actually role play a realistic scene in the dental office; and (3) observe the feedback you receive from others as they respond to your communication choices. Use the following chapter activities to review your understanding of the areas discussed in this chapter.

CHAPTER ACTIVITIES

1. In brief phrases, distinguish between verbal, vocal, and nonverbal–nonvocal communication.
2. Give a one-sentence illustration of each of these vocal aspects of com-

munication: volume, tonal quality, pitch, articulation, rate, pronunciation.

3. With a classmate, role play a telephone call to a dental office. Be realistic. If a tape recorder is available, record the conversation, then play it back to listen for vocal and verbal aspects of communication such as connotative and denotative meanings, emphasis and variety in pitch, rate, and clarity in articulation.

4. If you are in school where a dental clinic is a part of your training, ask another dental auxiliary to allow you to be a silent observer. Remain out of direct eyesight of the patient and take notes on nonverbal behavior. See if you can identify as many of the eight different forms of nonverbal communication as are described in this chapter. Note any others you may see which would fit aspects not mentioned in this chapter.

5. If you have access to videotape recording equipment, ask the operator of this equipment if you can record 20 minutes of role playing, and spend the remainder of the hour watching the playback. If this is possible, try the following exercise: Place a chair with its back facing the camera (this will be the dental chair). With the tape in record mode, walk toward the chair as if you were approaching a patient. Stand or sit as you would do in a normal dental operatory. Practice taking a medical and dental history with an imaginary patient (or use a classmate for more realistic role playing). Next, go through all the motions you can imagine that would occur during a dental examination involving you as either a dental assistant or a dental hygienist. Next, imagine that the dental care is complete and act out your parting movements and conversation with the "patient." When you are done, watch the playback of the videotape at least twice to observe your verbal, vocal, and nonverbal–nonvocal communication. (NOTE: Ask the camera operator to get closeups of your facial expressions and hand movements from time to time, as well as some medium shots and long shots; let the camera operator be creative to capture significant movements.)

REFERENCES

1. In Harold Stahmer, *Speak That I May See Thee!* (New York: Macmillan, 1968), p. 183.

2. Lane Cooper, *The Rhetoric of Aristotle*, trans. Lane Cooper (New York: Appleton-Century-Crofts, 1932), pp. 8, 131–40.

3. For a more current study of trust, see W. Barnett Pearce, "Trust in Interpersonal Communication," *Speech Monographs*, 41 (August 1974), 236–44.

4. The soldier's argument is an "either/or" fallacy—"either the tooth is pulled or it will be painful." It is a fallacy because there are more than two possibilities. (A root

canal is a third possibility.) Any current college textbook on speech communication or public address will provide a good definition of inductive and deductive reasoning. A good reference for understanding logic is W. Ward Fearnside and William B. Holther, *Fallacy: The Counterfeit of Argument* (Englewood Cliffs, N.J.: Prentice-Hall, 1959).

5. Peter B. Denes and Elliot N. Pinson, *The Speech Chain* (Bell Telephone Laboratories, 1963), p. 4.

6. For further study, see S. I. Hayakawa, *Language in Thought and Action,* 3rd ed. (New York: Harcourt Brace Jovanovich, 1972).

7. A contemporary discussion of acceptable American speech is in Stuart W. Hyde, *Television and Radio Announcing,* 3rd ed. (Boston: Houghton Mifflin, 1979), Chapter 7, "American English Usage," and Chapter 8, "The New Language."

8. For further reading in nonverbal communication, see Ray T. Birdwhistell, *Kinesics and Context* (New York: Ballantine Books, 1970); Edward T. Hall, *The Silent Language* (New York: Doubleday, 1959); and Jurgen Ruesch, *Nonverbal Communication* (Berkeley: University of California Press, 1956).

9. J. J. Edney, "Place and Space: The Effects of Experience with a Physical Locale," *Journal of Experimental and Social Psychology,* 8, no. 2 (1972) 124–35.

10. Hall, *The Silent Language,* pp. 15–30.

BIBLIOGRAPHY

ARGYLE, MICHAEL, *The Psychology of Interpersonal Behavior.* Baltimore: Penguin Books, 1972.

BERGER, CHARLES R., and CALABRESE, RICHARD J., "Some Explorations in Initial Interaction and Beyond: Toward a Developmental Theory of Interpersonal Communication," *Human Communication Research,* I, no. 2 (Winter 1975).

BIRDWHISTELL, RAY L., *Kinesics and Context.* New York: Ballantine Books, 1970.

BROOKS, WILLIAM D., *Speech Communication,* 3rd ed., Dubuque, Ia.: W. C. Brown, 1976.

BROOKS, WILLIAM D., and EMMERT, PHILLIP, *Interpersonal Communication,* 2nd ed. Dubuque, Ia.: W. C. Brown, 1976.

COOPER, LANE, *The Rhetoric of Aristotle.* New York: Appleton-Century-Crofts, 1932.

DENES, PETER, and PINSON, ELLIOT N., *The Speech Chain.* Bell Telephone Laboratories, 1963.

EDNEY, J. J., "Place and Space: The Effects of Experience with a Physical Locale," *Journal of Experimental and Social Psychology,* 8, no. 2 (1972), 124–35.

FEARNSIDE, W. WARD, and HOLTHER, WILLIAM B., *Fallacy: The Counterfeit of Argument.* Englewood Cliffs, N.J.: Prentice-Hall, 1959.

GOULDING, PETER C., "What the Public Thinks of the Dentist and Dental Health," *Journal of the American Dental Association,* 70 (May 1965).

GREENBERG, JOEL, "Why I Hate the Dentist," *Science News,* 112, (September 1977), 170.

HALL, EDWARD T., *The Silent Language.* New York: Doubleday, 1959.

HAYAKAWA, S. I., *Language in Thought and Action*, 3rd ed. New York: Harcourt Brace Jovanovich, 1972.

HYDE, STUART W., *Television and Radio Announcing*, 3rd ed. Boston: Houghton Mifflin, 1979.

MARSE, BEN W., and PHELPS, LYNN A., *Interpersonal Communication: A Relational Perspective*. Minneapolis: Burgess, 1980.

PEARCE, W., BARNETT, "Trust in Interpersonal Communication," *Speech Monographs*, 41 (August 1974), 236–44.

POWELL, JOHN, S. J., *Fully Human, Fully Alive*. Niles, Ill.: Argus Communications, 1969.

REID, CLYDE, *The Empty Pulpit*. New York: Harper & Row, 1967.

ROGERS, CARL, "The Characteristics of a Helping Relationship." Paper delivered at the APGA Convention, St. Louis, Miss., March 31–April 3, 1958.

ROKEACH, MILTON, "Long Range Experimental Modification of Values, Attitudes, and Behavior." Paper presented as part of a symposium, *Human Behavior and Its Control*, American Association for the Advancement of Science, Chicago, Ill., 1970.

RUESCH, JURGEN, *Nonverbal Communication*. Berkeley: University of California Press, 1956.

TOCH, HANS, and MACLEAN, MALCOLM S., JR., "Perception, Communication and Educational Research: A Transactional View," *Audio Visual Communication Review*, X (1962).

SAKUMURA, JOSEPH S., "Values of Dental Hygiene Faculty and Students," *Educational Directions*, 2, no. 2 (May 1977), 6–8.

SEBALD, HANS, "Limitations of Communication: Mechanisms of Image Maintenance in Form of Selective Perception; Selective Memory and Selective Distortion," *Journal of Communication*, XII (September 1962).

SHERWOOD, JOHN J., "Self-Identity and Referent Others," *Sociemetry*, 28 (1965).

STAHMER, HAROLD, *Speak That I May See Thee!* New York: Macmillan, 1968, p. 183.

WATZLAWICK, PAUL, BEAVIN, JANET HELMICK, and JACKSON, DON D., *Pragmatics of Human Communication*. New York: W. W. Norton, 1967.

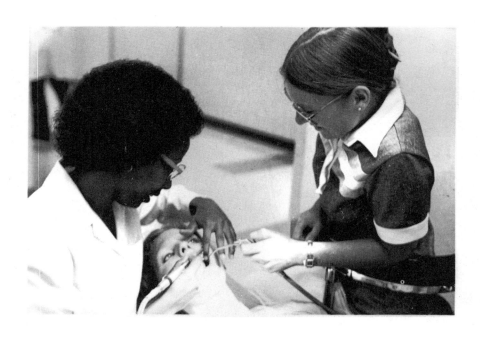

PROFESSIONAL ASPECTS OF COMMUNICATION

> *In school, I never thought about the importance of communication. It was not until I actually went to work in a dental office that I realized how important communication skills are in dentistry.*

A Certified Dental Assistant

KEY POINTS

CHAPTER 6
Preparing for First Impressions
  physical environment
  interpersonal encounter
Communication Review

CHAPTER 7
Interviewing Techniques
  open-ended questions
  closed questions
  repetition
  interpretive or clarifying
    responses
  probing responses
  leading questions
  nonverbal encouragement
  summarizing
  paraphrasing
  closure

Listening
  problems
  skills
Evaluating Patient Responses

CHAPTER 8
Theories of Learning
  satisfying needs
  behavior management
  competency
  fear reduction
Two Learning Approaches
  deductive
  inductive
Motivation
  definition
  theories
  attitude and behavior change
Persuasion
  definition
  guidelines for persuasive
    communication

First Impressions

6

The first time you meet a new patient, chances are that your communication skills will be tested before your technical/dental skills are put into practice. And each time thereafter the initial contact between you and a returning patient will either reinforce or alter those earliest impressions. These first impressions and initial contacts set the mood for all that follows as you begin to work with the patient toward preventive dental care.

Following are two stories told by dental auxiliaries:

In walked this big, strong army corporal who said he'd never been to a dentist before. The only time anyone in his family had ever gone to a dentist it was to have an aching tooth pulled. He was in pain and the expression on his face told me he was scared to death just to sit down in the dental chair. In his mind, he knew he'd have to have his tooth extracted. The doctor had been running patients through the clinic so fast that sometimes he would have them in the chair only long enough to yank out their tooth, sometimes before the anesthetic had made them numb. This guy was so scared I needed time to calm him down and talk to him before the doctor saw him. Fortunately, I did get him calmed down and, as it turned out, he didn't have to lose his tooth. He probably won't be so afraid next time.

A Certified Dental Assistant in an army-camp dental clinic

111

I had a patient who was so nervous that he pulled up his knees so that his feet were flat on the footrest and he constantly banged his knees together. His wife had to come into the operatory to help him make decisions.

A Registered Dental Hygienist in private practice

In what ways might you have dealt with either of these cases? What are your verbal, vocal, and nonverbal–nonvocal communication choices? What is your perception of each of the people described? What roles do you find in these stories? All that was described in the first five chapters comes into play when a real-life situation confronts you in a clinic or dental office. To give yourself a trial run, try the following communication exercises so as to get a feel for how you might deal with similar situations.

COMMUNICATION EXERCISE 6–1

Analyze the CDA's patient (first example) and give your response.

What did the patient's physical appearance say to the CDA?

What was the first impression given to the CDA by the patient's physical appearance?

In what ways did his verbal communication contradict or reinforce his non-verbal message?

Verbally, what would you say to this patient under these conditions? (Write this out in complete sentences, just as you would talk to him.)

Describe briefly the following vocal and nonverbal choices:
Your tone of voice

Your rate of speaking

Your eye contact

COMMUNICATION EXERCISE 6–2

Analyze the RDH's situation (second example) and give your response.

What might this patient's body movements indicate?

What silent message might the wife's presence give?

What would be your initial comments and to whom would these be directed?

PREPARING FOR FIRST IMPRESSIONS

In the two examples described above, the dental auxiliaries faced unusual circumstances. Under ordinary daily preventive-care circumstances in a dental clinic or office, you will meet people having a variety of backgrounds, dental experiences, and established expectations and stereotypes about you as a dental auxiliary. They come to you with different needs and emotions. Because your initial contact with them is crucial to setting the mood for all subsequent communication and preventive dental care, it is important to prepare and be ready for them.

If, in fact, your communication skills determine the climate in which you practice your technical dental skills, then it is worth taking seriously two factors which influence the first impressions and initial contact. These factors,

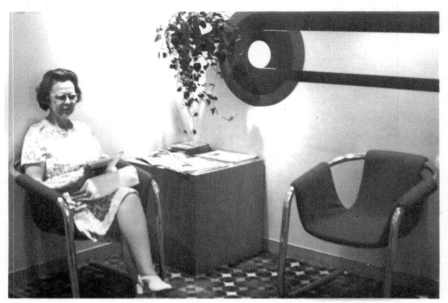

Figure 6–1. The waiting room of a dental office is one of the first places where patients develop their first impressions. Here, one waiting room was designed for a general practice and the other (Fig. 6–2) was specifically created for a pedodontic office.

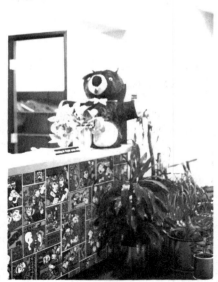

Figure 6–2.

which have been discussed in preceding chapters, are (1) the physical environment and (2) the interpersonal encounter. There are ways to prepare for each of these factors.

The Physical Environment

THE WAITING ROOM.   The two places where the environment influences the patient most by setting the emotional climate for preventive dental care are the waiting room and the operatory. You yourself may spend virtually no time in the waiting room—yet consider the effect on a patient waiting as long as 15 minutes in a waiting room that is a comfortable and pleasant place. This place introduces a first-time patient to your place of work. It is also a visible reminder for returning patients, reminding them of all that has happened in previous visits, both pleasant and unpleasant. If the waiting area is neatly arranged in an uncrowded manner, with pleasing colors on walls, lighting that is not harsh, and reading material selected with patients' general interests in mind, they will be in a comfortable and relaxing environment. Cleanliness is important, also. Background music should not be loud or offensive. Pedodontic offices might have a few sturdy toys, children's books and perhaps a television set tuned to a channel suitable for preteens (such as the Public Broadcasting System). You can have some influence on the neatness of the room, either by calling attention to it in staff meetings or by being responsible for it yourself.

The best way to check out this part of the physical environment is to take a few minutes to go to the waiting room and sit there, observing it as would any patient at any time of day. Suppose you had to wait there for at least 15 minutes, anticipating a periodontal checkup or waiting for oral surgery. Would the room be a comfortable and pleasant place to wait? What do you see? How comfortable are the chairs? What kinds of talk do you hear in the receptionist's area? Does the receptionist have a pleasant tone of voice in the regular course of business? Is there personal talk, perhaps confidential information that is too easily overheard, regarding finances or other matters relating to patients? How is the lighting? Would you be interested in any of the magazines available in the room? Overall, how do you feel? It is important for you to know this in order to see how patients are introduced to the office or clinic in which you work.

THE OPERATORY.   Next, walk into the operatory, sit in the dental chair, and look around. Does it seem like a comfortable and pleasant setting? Is it neat and clean? Does it smell clean? The way you feel is similar to the way patients will feel in this environment. If there is background music, is the volume low and is the style of music appropriate? Patients who are in middle and late

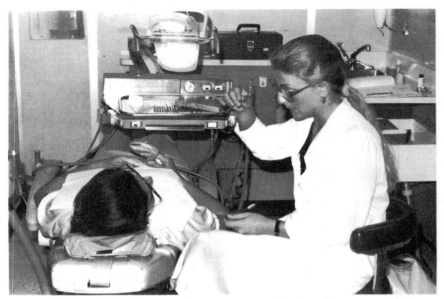

Figure 6-3. Notice the neatness and attractiveness of the dental instruments in Figure 6-3 and the pleasant view in Figure 6-4. The arrangement of the environment adds to a positive perception by patients.

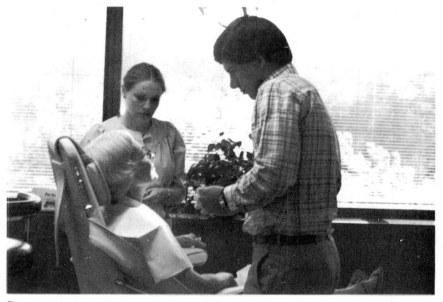

Figure 6-4.

adolescence may prefer higher amplitude and currently popular music, while younger and older patients tend to prefer background music which is simply that—background. The purpose is to calm and relax a patient, not to add complications to the dental appointment. Knowing your patient is the key to designing the most appropriate environment.

The Interpersonal Encounter

THE RECEPTIONIST'S ROLE. When a patient enters a dental clinic or dental office, the first person he or she encounters is usually the receptionist. If you are this person or if you are asked to train this person, be aware that the receptionist can set an emotional mood with the patient in many ways. Verbally, the words used should show respect and interest in the patient. Vocally, the sound of the receptionist's voice, both over the telephone and in person, should be pleasant. Indifference to these speech habits can make a difference between a defensive or a cooperative patient, one who feels free to talk or one who is closed. Nonverbal behavior also is important for first impressions, including one's dress, facial expressions, eye contact, and the individualized attention the patient receives.

A receptionist at an urban clinic was observed answering a question posed by a new patient: "How do I get to the doctor's room?" asked the patient. The receptionist stood up, took off her glasses, and started to clean them, looked away from the patient, and with a rather snobbish voice said, "Ya follow the red dots." The receptionist's manner and tone of voice made the patient feel that her question had been stupid. She was so intimidated that she went to ask another waiting patient what the "red dots" were, not knowing that they marked a directional path on the floor. The patient seemed isolated and confused, alone in a strange place full of busy people and receiving a message of indifference from the receptionist; this was not a very helpful and positive introduction to the clinic.

COMMUNICATION EXERCISE 6-3

Write in the space below what your communication choices would be if you were the receptionist or if you were to train the receptionist in proper "first-impression" communication:

Nonverbal choices (eye contact, posture, gestures)

(continued)

COMMUNICATION EXERCISE 6-3 *(Contd)*

Vocal choices (pitch, rate, volume)

Verbal choices (words, connotation, denotation)

THE DENTAL AUXILIARY'S ROLE.   In the actual situation described above, it was a Certified Dental Assistant's task to overcome the receptionist's mistake. The CDA's response was to smile, look the patient in the eyes, and with a conversational volume, rate, and pitch to her voice say, "Hi Mrs. M_____, I'm Jill. Will you come this way, please?" The pleasant, personal approach of the dental assistant helped to overcome what had happened in the waiting room. The frown on the patient's face changed to a smile, clear feedback that the dental assistant had made the right choices.

A normal social greeting, including names, is an acceptable way to begin. Eye contact is important. A handshake is not necessary and is usually not considered to be appropriate in professional dental situations. Simple verbal directions are important. What you may take for granted may be just the thing a patient needs to know, including such simple phrases as "Please follow me" or "Please be seated (in the dental chair)," and "Would you rest your head back, please?"

Throughout these ritualistic procedures of getting the patient from the waiting area to the operatory and into the dental chair, your tone of voice, gentleness of touch, and careful arrangement of items in the operatory will set the mood for the communication and dental procedures that follow. Your own physical appearance as well as that of the surrounding environment contribute to the total interpersonal communication which affects both your interviewing and your dental-care procedures.

CHECKLIST OF COMMUNICATION SKILLS.   Although it is often the role of a dentist or a personnel director to hire receptionists, you, as a dental auxiliary, may be asked to make suggestions or participate in the selection of a new receptionist. Here is a brief checklist of communication skills you could use:

Telephone Voice	Clear articulation, pleasant tone, adequate volume.
Verbal Communication	Standard American English vocabulary, good grammar, absence of popular slang; ability to ask basic questions and give clear instructions.
Physical Behavior	Neat, clean appearance; good eye contact while speaking and listening.

Self-Concept	Confident in ability to do the work; confident in ability to communicate with people from a wide variety of racial, ethnic, socioeconomic, and educational backgrounds; nondefensive with angry or emotional people; at ease with people of all ages, from early childhood through old age.
Role Concept	Ability to work as team member with others on dental team rather than as an isolated individual working autonomously; ability to see role as part of total preventive dental care of patients; willing to care for physical environment of waiting room and receptionist's area.

Because receptionists in larger offices and clinics are rarely seen in the operatory, the rest of the dental team may not be aware of their roles in the entire process of the patient's entry and departure; the receptionist gives the first and last impression at your office or clinic.

Unless you also serve as a receptionist—which CDAs and RDHs sometimes do in private practices—you are the next person to greet the patient. And you are one of the dental professionals whom a patient perceives as part of the "serious part" of the visit.

THE PATIENT'S EXPECTATIONS.   The patient arrives with assumptions about what will happen. Some of these assumptions are based on past experience and are likely to be correct. Others may be based on preconceived ideas given them by friends' stories and their own past experiences which are different than what they are about to experience. They may assume that their teeth are O.K. and not be expecting any problems. Or they may expect to experience pain, embarrassment, or a number of other feelings which relate to past visits to dental offices. Also, they likely come with a stereotype about dental auxiliaries and dentists. In some ways, stereotypes may be helpful to you if they reinforce your effort to be a careful, honest professional interested in the patient's preventive dental care. On the other hand, stereotypes can also be harmful to the relationship because they can create expectations that are not realistic.

What helps first is your own self-concept and your own clear identity about your role. Confidence in your medical and dental knowledge and ability to do the skills required in the dental operatory is important to develop a strong self-concept as a dental auxiliary. This will be reflected in your verbal, vocal, and nonverbal communication with individual patients, and they will see it.

Preparing for first impressions probably is more complex than the actual interpersonal encounter itself. Your attitude and the dental environment are two factors that must be "ready" ahead of time. The initial contact can be as simple as this:

> "Good morning, Mrs. _____; it's good to see you again."
> "Mr. _____, the last door to the left, please."
> "Hi, Joanie, how are you this afternoon? Have you been having any problems since the last time you were here?"

Such simple, natural-sounding introductions and welcomes may or may not elicit equally easy responses from the patient. Remember, this is your territory, not the patient's, and any uneasiness present will be the patient's, not yours (assuming you have a confident self-image). So you may get such responses as:

> (Silence; a weak smile.)
> "Hello"
> "Uh-huh."
> "I'm fine; how are you?"
> "I'm O.K. (but I wish I weren't here, says the tone of voice)."

You may notice that the patient is communicating with various degrees of openness and defensiveness. If patients talk very little, it is likely that they are more apprehensive and are pulling into themselves for defense. But a very talkative person may also be using speech to cope with anxiety or even fear. It is important to remember that you are in charge and the patient will appreciate any polite, gentle, and clear directions or requests you make at this early stage.

In order to prepare for the interpersonal aspect of your initial contact with patients, let's review the variables mentioned in the first five chapters, keeping in mind the two situations described at the beginning of this chapter.

COMMUNICATION REVIEW QUESTIONS

1. What is your perception of yourself? Of the patient? Of others in the room?
2. How do you see the role of yourself as a professional person? The patient's role? The role of others in the room?
3. What might be your verbal communication choices: Is your vocabulary technical/dental/medical, or conversational? Is your vocabulary con-

notative or denotative? Is your vocabulary accurate, appropriate, and concise? Is your vocabulary informative, instructive, or persuasive?

4. What might be your vocal communication choices? Consider the following: Volume/amplitude/loudness; pitch; rate; authoritative/direct manner; calm/patient/understanding attitude; articulation clear and distinct pronunciation.

SUMMARY

In this brief chapter, we have discussed some of the basic aspects of patients and dental auxiliaries meeting for the first time in a dental setting. The two main considerations in this context are the physical environment and the interpersonal encounter. The two most significant environmental influences on a patient's first impressions occur in the waiting room and the dental operatory. The waiting room introduces a first-time patient to the auxiliary's place of work; for a return patient it reinforces initial impressions, and reminds the patient of all that has happened here in previous appointments. Nonverbally it is saying a great deal to patients, and attention to the arrangement of the room, the colors, the lighting, and reading material, as well as the cleanliness, are vital. The purpose is to help calm and relax the patient. The interpersonal encounter between the patient and the dental office is a vital link for all that follows as the auxiliary begins to work with the patient toward preventive dental care. Verbal, vocal, and nonverbal communication choices selected by the patient begin to create first impressions. The receptionist has a big influence on a patient's first impressions. Communication skills to be considered are telephone voice, verbal communication, physical behavior, self-concept, and role concept. It is important to remember that patients arrive at the dental office with a set of assumptions about the environment and what will happen in the environment. The dental auxiliary's interpersonal encounter with the patient becomes even more important in a consideration of the development of first impressions. Therefore, it is useful for the auxiliary to ask questions like: What is my perception of my role, the patient's role, and the role of others in the office? How do I see myself as a professional person? What are the roles of the other dental health team members? What are my most-used verbal communication choices? The patient's first impressions about the dental office, and the first impressions of the dental staff concerning the patient, are significant in the successful rendering of preventive dental care.

CHAPTER ACTIVITIES

1. State the two factors cited in this chapter which influence first impressions in an initial contact.

2. What are the two main locations in which a patient receives and decodes nonverbal messages about the dental environment?

3. Visit a reception area or waiting room (or close your eyes and visualize the last one you sat in) and on paper draw a floor plan of the room. Include furniture and location of the receptionist's desk. Make notations about colors, sounds, odors, neatness, cleanliness, and comfort. Note any other sensory receptions that influence your perception of the room. State how this place makes you feel.

4. List five changes you would make in the waiting room described in the previous exercise. Explain why these changes would be beneficial to a patient who may wait there for at least 15 minutes.

5. Write a hypothetical "script" for an initial interpersonal communication event between yourself as a dental auxiliary and a new patient.

6. Write a list of communication skills you would look for if you were to interview an applicant for receptionist in your office.

Interviewing, Listening, and Evaluating Responses

7

The two most verbal interpersonal situations in a dental office occur when you talk with a patient in initial interviews and when you talk with members of the staff. Of all the times when communication will be used in a dental office, those when you interview a patient in the operatory may be when verbal skills are most frequently used.

Just as learning a basic communication model (Chapter 2) can help you analyze and understand every communication event, learning basic interviewing skills will apply to almost every interviewing situation.

Interviewing takes many forms according to the main goal of the situation. Interviews can be for the purposes of employment, personal counseling, obtaining journalistic information, market research and opinion sampling, and obtaining medical/dental histories. The latter is what you will find most helpful in your work.

Because interviewing requires both speaking and listening skills, the following information will give you some basic facts concerning (1) eliciting information by using specific techniques; (2) the art of good listening; and (3) the interviewee's responses.

INTERVIEWING

Dental interviews are usually for the purpose of obtaining factual information. However, as the sample interview following will show, obtaining such information requires more than just asking for it in the way you would call up information on a computer terminal. Obtaining even the most basic information from another human being requires that you are able to ask questions in a variety of ways and apply other decoding and encoding skills as required.

Goals

To apply the familiar words of management to interviewing, interviews have basic *goals* and *objectives*. The overall goal is to obtain information helpful to the delivery of preventive dental health care of the patient. The objectives are like stair steps, one leading to the other, as the following list shows.

>   5. Formulate procedures for preventive dental care
>   4. Evaluate Step 3
>   3. Analyze Steps 1 and 2
> 2. Describe dental/medical history
> 1. Identify reason for the appointment

Steps 1 and 2 are those which involve basic interviewing and listening skills. Steps 3, 4, and 5 are, by law, reserved for the dentist and will not be covered in this book. We will be concerned with the first two steps as they occur in interviewing.

Interviewing Techniques

The types of interview techniques used to elicit patient information, frequently referred to as types of "questions," are more accurately described as a combination of verbal and/or vocal encoding. Ten types of techniques most often used in this situation are (1) open-ended questions, (2) closed questions, (3) repetition, (4) interpretative or clarifying responses, (5) probing responses, (6) leading questions or statements, (7) nonverbal encouragement, (8) summarizing, (9) paraphrasing, and (10) closure. It will help you to learn each type and then to practice each with a friend or classmate. Interviewing is an art, learned best through practice.

OPEN-ENDED QUESTIONS.   This technique allows the interviewee to respond in any way he or she chooses. Not only do you leave the verbal door open for the interviewee, but you leave your own mind open for any response. No assumptions are made about what kind of answer is appropriate. "How are

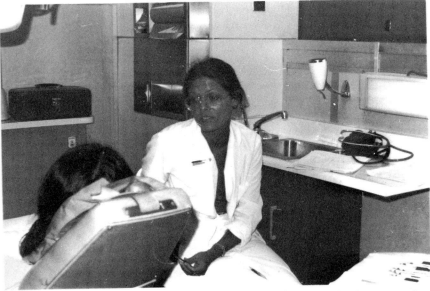

Figure 7–1. The interviewing process is a multifaceted communication encounter. Facial expressions, eye contact, and proximity, as well as the words you use, are important in interviewing. See also Figure 7–2.

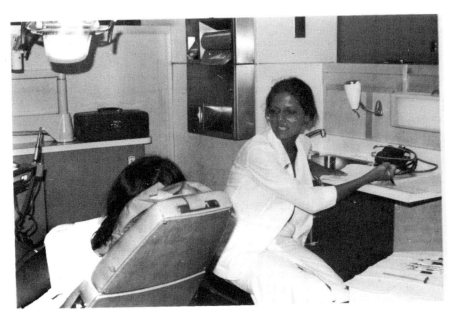

Figure 7–2.

you today, Mrs. _____?" is open but possibly too general for a realistic response. Yet such a question could lead to interesting responses if the patient either has special dental concerns to discuss or has personal needs to talk with someone. If a patient responded, "Oh, I've been having a little problem in the back when I chew," you could ask an open-ended question like, "What kinds of specific problems have you noticed?"

CLOSED QUESTIONS.   Such questions ask for specific information and usually begin with such words as "What," "When," "Is," "Do," "Does," "Are," "Who," "Where," and "Will." Closed questions can be answered with either a "yes" or "no" response. If you need to know information that can be answered by a yes, or no, or a short "statistical-type" response, then a closed question is what you should use. However, inexperienced interviewers often *expect* a detailed answer when they ask a closed question, only to receive a quick one-word answer. In such a case, open-ended questions are better. Here are some typical closed questions:

> "When was the last time you had a checkup?"
> "Do you floss?"
> "Who is your medical doctor?"
> "Where do you notice the pain?"
> "Is this tender when I touch it?"

During an interview for a medical/dental history, many questions are of the closed-question type.

REPETITION.   When you use repetition, you are trying to make sure you heard the response correctly, not showing surprise or judgment. You are try-ing to find out if you have decoded the information correctly. On a dental history form you want to be accurate, so repeating information for your own assurance is a safeguard. A patient may mumble, turn away while answering, or not articulate clearly. Repeating the patient's age, medication, diseases, and other relevant information aids accuracy.

INTERPRETATIVE OR CLARIFYING RESPONSES.   These are statements which you, the interviewer, make in order to make sure that you understand more com-plex responses. With such a statement, you are actually entering further into a dialogue form of interpersonal communication, as described in Chapter 2, which may eventually lead to analysis, evaluation, and the action necessary for preventive dentistry. An interpretative response might follow a closed question, like this:

Q: Did you have any childhood diseases?
A: I'm not sure what you mean.
Q: Like measles, chicken pox, and so forth.

Or, it could follow an open-ended question like this:

Q: Tell me a little about any hospital visits you've had.
A: You mean like when I had my baby?
Q: Yes, or any time you went for tests, treatment for special problems, or surgery.

A clarifying response or question is one that simply asks for the interviewee to explain an answer further:

Q: Do you floss regularly?
A: Oh, I guess, sometimes.
Q: Would you say once a week, every other day or . . . ?
A: When I think about it.
Q: Would you say you floss regularly or infrequently?
A: I'd say infrequently, maybe once or twice a month.

Interpretative and clarifying responses such as these provide both interviewer and interviewee with feedback each needs in order to move from general to specific information and clearer understanding of the meaning of the information.

PROBING RESPONSES.   The technique of making probing responses is similar to interpretative and clarifying statements in that they seek more information. While the clarifying statement is used as the interviewer seeks to understand what a previous statement meant, a probing response tries to get deeper into the details and perhaps the reasons behind the details. A simple statement on your part like, "Tell me more about that," keeps the patient on the same topic but asks for elaboration. In this case, the probe takes the form of an open-ended question, allowing the patient to keep talking in any way he or she chooses, although the patient is expected to remain on the same topic. "Oh, really?" and "That's interesting, tell me more," are other probing responses to an interviewee's statement.

LEADING QUESTIONS OR STATEMENTS.   These guide the response of the patient and should be used sparingly until you are looking for specific information which other kinds of interviewing techniques have not elicited. Here's an example in a conversation with a teenage patient:

Q: Do you have a lot of sugar in your diet?
A: I wouldn't say so.

Q: Well, like soda pop or candy bars—do you drink a lot of soda pop for example?

A: Oh, sure, every day; a lot.

A couple of cautions about leading questions are that they should not be used extensively at the expense of other kinds, because they tend to guide the interviewee down a narrow path of what you are looking for, putting words into the patient's mouth, which may result in your missing other information that could have been elicited had you allowed the patient to be more self-disclosing. Second, such questions can become judgmental comments on your part, denoting your own values or desires for the patient's behavior.

For example, a dental hygienist asked an adolescent what kind of musical instrument he was learning to play. When the youth answered that he was learning to play the clarinet, the RDH's voice took on a judgmental, almost angry tone, when she responded, "You're not going to play something like *that* with an overbite like you have, are you? Couldn't you choose a violin or something?" This kind of judgment has no place in a dental or medical interview, no matter how well-intended.

NONVERBAL ENCOURAGEMENT.   This method of eliciting information can be either vocal or nonvocal. It is a form of probing and clarifying. If you wish to encourage a patient to keep on talking about a particular matter, your silence will allow him or her to keep talking. Silence and a nod of the head is an easy way of encouraging an interviewee to keep going. Or a simple vocal sound, such as "Uh-huh" or "Mmmm," followed by a smile or a nod while maintaining good eye contact, will let the patient know that you are listening and are interested in hearing more. The less you talk, the more freedom the other person has to open up, go into more detail, and verbalize his or her thoughts.

SUMMARIZING.   In this technique you do most of the talking; you make a verbal listing of what you believe you have heard throughout an interview or during a lengthy portion of an interview. You probably would not take time to summarize all of a patient's factual medical and dental history. However, you may wish to summarize some of the noticeable highlights of those facts which a patient has felt to be significant. This is a way of letting a patient know what you have heard. It has an added benefit of letting the patient know that you feel he or she is an important person because you have, indeed, listened carefully to what the interviewee has told you.

PARAPHRASING.   Paraphrasing is putting into your own words what you have heard the interviewee say. It is similar to clarifying because it is a way of helping both of you understand that you are in mutual agreement about what has been said. If the patient responds, "Yes, that's what I said," or "Yes, that is what I was trying to tell you," then you know you did understand, and the patient feels comfortable in knowing that you do understand. Paraphrasing is a form of feedback from you to the patient, letting him or her know that you have decoded what had been encoded. It is usually important to paraphrase after a rather complicated response by the patient or after an awkward attempt has been made by the patient to explain something which he or she may feel is unclear. Here is an example:

PATIENT: Well, my neighbor keeps telling me that coffee and cigarettes will stain your teeth and she may be right, you know, because I don't seem to be able to keep my teeth as white as I'd like.

DENTAL
AUXILIARY: You feel that it is drinking coffee and smoking that causes the stain on your teeth?

PATIENT: Yes, I think so. That's right.

CLOSURE.   This is what you do to bring the interview to an end. You can use verbal, vocal, and nonverbal–nonvocal means to accomplish closure. Putting down your pen and clipboard, standing up, smiling, raising or dropping the pitch of your voice and saying, "Thank you" can be sufficient. Simple interviews, taking only a few minutes, are usually easy to close. Long ones, in which the patient has been encouraged to talk more freely, may require more assertiveness on your part. You may need to decide whether a talkative patient has therapeutic needs to talk to you, which lonely people or people with pressing personal problems may often need to do; or they may be using long conversation to avoid the actual forthcoming dental work. Perhaps they just want to be sociable. You need to decide when it is appropriate to let a patient talk beyond your own needs for information. Still, you can terminate the interview by saying, "Thank you for helping me answer these questions. If you'll rest your head back now and open your mouth, we'll take a look at your teeth." This can be said without "putting down" the patient or even cutting off his or her talk. You may still allow the patient to talk, of course, after the interview is completed, if there is time between the interview and subsequent dental procedures. However, with closure, you have clearly stated that the dental/medical interview portion of the appointment is terminated. If nothing else follows, you can say something like, "You've had a lot to share with me today, Mr. _____. I'll be seeing you in ten days. Thank you for coming in." If a patient persists in conversation and you wish to terminate the appointment, you can start toward the operatory door, wait momentarily for the patient to follow, then walk to the receptionist's desk and talk to the receptionist about the time and date of the patient's next appointment. Closure can be, "Thank you Mr. _____. We'll see you in ten days," followed by a smile and then by your return to the operatory.

TWO TYPICAL INTERVIEWS

In dental interviewing there are brief interviews and there are more complete interviews, the latter taken when a new patient begins with a clinic or office. Dental-school clinics also require lengthy, detailed medical and dental histories which require longer interviews. Following are two typical interviews. The first is brief and could occur when a patient is returning to his or her regular dental office for a six-month checkup. The second is a portion of a more lengthy interview. As you read these interviews, notice in the right-hand column the types of questions being asked, as well as other information. You may wish to try to identify these yourself by covering the right-hand column as you read.

INTERVIEW PRECEDING SIX-MONTH CHECKUP

DENTAL AUXILIARY: Good morning, Mrs. _____. Good to see you. Have you been to the hospital since I saw you last? — Closed question

PATIENT: No.

AUXILIARY: Are you on any medications? — Closed question

PATIENT: Yes, I am.

AUXILIARY: What medications are you on now? — Closed question

PATIENT: (Gives names of medications.)

AUXILIARY: Who is your physician? — Closed question

PATIENT: (Gives name of physician.)

AUXILIARY: Do you have any contagious diseases? — Closed question

PATIENT: No, thank goodness.

AUXILIARY: O.K. Now, let's take your blood pressure. After that I will palpate your gums for an oral cancer examination. — Interpretation. Then we'll clean and polish your teeth, O.K.? — Closed question

PATIENT: O.K.

INTERVIEW FOR MORE COMPLETE DATA

DENTAL AUXILIARY: Good afternoon, Mrs. _____. My name is Judy. Is this your first visit to the clinic? — Closed question

PATIENT: No. Well, yes, recently, it is. I used to come here; but that was several years ago.

AUXILIARY: This is your first visit in several years? — Paraphrase

PATIENT: Yes, you might say that. (Laughs.) My husband will probably come in sometime too, one of these days.

AUXILIARY: Mrs. _____, first we like to get a medical and dental history when a patient is either here for the first time or, like you, is returning after a few years. So, I'd like to ask you some questions about your medical and dental background. Your age is . . . — Closed question

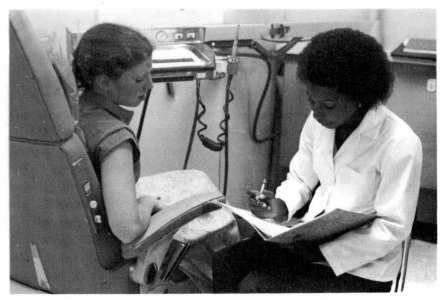

Figure 7–3. Interviewing is an important step in getting to know your patient.

PATIENT:	I'm 73.	
AUXILIARY:	And your husband's name . . .	Closed, recalls earlier information
PATIENT:	(Gives full name of husband.)	
AUXILIARY:	Any childhood diseases?	Closed; not specific
PATIENT:	Yes.	
AUXILIARY:	All of them?	Leading question; fails to elicit specific data
PATIENT:	Yes.	
AUXILIARY:	Tell me a little about any hospital visits you've had.	Open-ended and leading
PATIENT:	Just once, when I had my daughter. I've been pretty healthy, I guess.	
AUXILIARY:	Any broken bones?	Closed but unclear (does she mean past or present?)
PATIENT:	No.	
AUXILIARY:	You're lucky. I've had one. Have you had any problems with your heart, liver, kidneys or other organs?	Humanizing comment breaks monotony of the questionnaire Closed question
PATIENT:	Well, I may have had a heart murmur several years ago. I don't know for sure.	

AUXILIARY: Has there been any heart-related illness in your family?	Closed question
PATIENT: My father died of a heart attack at the age of 83.	
AUXILIARY: No other problems with kidney, lungs, blood pressure or anything like that?	Clarifying question
PATIENT: No.	
AUXILIARY: Tell me more about the heart murmur.	Probing statement
PATIENT: The doctor thought I may have had one but he couldn't diagnose it for sure.	
AUXILIARY: (Silent. Maintains eye contact with patient.)	Encouraging nonverbal behavior
PATIENT: I'm not clear about it. It was two years ago.	
AUXILIARY: Would you mind if we call your physician on this, just as a precaution?	Closed question
PATIENT: No. That's fine.	
AUXILIARY: (Asks several related questions.)	
PATIENT: I feel like I'm going into the hospital!	
AUXILIARY: You think these forms are like the ones you might have to fill out if you were going into a hospital? We only have to do this this time; next time we won't need to go through such a long form. It's important to get this, especially to know what allergies a patient has or medications you might be using which would cause a problem when dental work is done. There's only one more page.	Paraphrase interpretation
PATIENT: (Smiles.)	
AUXILIARY: Have most of your visits to dentists been for checkups?	Leading question
PATIENT: Yes. I've had pretty good teeth. I still have them all!	
AUXILIARY: Tell me about what you do at home.	Open but unclear; hence, misunderstood by patient
PATIENT: Well, I sew and garden. I go bowling.	
AUXILIARY: Tell me about how you take care of your teeth.	Open-ended
PATIENT: Oh, I brush twice a day and floss at night.	
AUXILIARY: Could you tell me more, like about your diet?	Probing question
PATIENT: (Describes regular foods eaten.)	
AUXILIARY: Do you drink a lot of coffee?	Probing and closed
PATIENT: No.	
AUXILIARY: I drink tea a lot.	Probes by own self-disclosure
PATIENT: I do smoke about a pack of cigarettes a day.	
AUXILIARY: I'll bet you have the great American bathroom syndrome when you brush your teeth, don't you? (Smiling.) You brush your teeth with tooth-	Humor as a leading question

> paste in the bathroom at the sink with the water running.
> PATIENT: (Smiles and nods head, indicating "yes.")
> AUXILIARY: (Offers alternative ways of dental care, then continues interview for dental and medical history.)

As the words of both the dental auxiliary and the patient indicate, interviewing is a human activity which requires more than objective humorless technique. Rather, interviewing is one more way in which two human beings communicate, and it is important to remember that though the purpose of an interview may be simply for obtaining factual data for a written record, it need not be a mechanical process. Human sensitivity and empathy help to develop trust between interviewee and interviewer. Trust is the foundation on which all cooperative communication is built. Hence, the humanizing aspect of interviewing sets a constructive tone for all subsequent communication throughout preventive dental care with the patient.

LISTENING TO THE PATIENT

Closely related to what you say in interviewing is the listening you do. Listening obviously is important in interviewing and is equally important during all other stages of your work. Because we spend many of our waking hours listening, we may assume that there is nothing difficult about it and that there is nothing to learn about it. However, people do not always listen as well as we might assume and there are, in fact, many barriers to effective listening which require a conscious effort to overcome. It is possible to correct some of the problems that interfere with good listening.

Listening Problems

Listening problems that may occur in a dental setting usually involve one or more of the following: (1) noises, (2) patient behavior and appearance, (3) private agenda, (4) stereotypes, (5) selective listening, (6) speech habits, (7) role expectations, (8) defensiveness and silent arguing, and (9) impatience. Let us look at each of these.

NOISES. Interference of noise from machinery, sirens, traffic, airplanes, children screaming, others talking and phones ringing can cause you to be momentarily distracted from listening.

PATIENT'S BEHAVIOR AND APPEARANCE. A nervous or highly active patient may distract you visually from paying close attention audibly. Likewise, the way a person dresses, his or her natural physical attributes such as size, shape, and grooming can also be distracting, especially if you spend any time thinking about this while the person is talking. Persons with physical impairments can cause you to listen carelessly. People of different nationality from your own may dress or behave differently than those with whom you are socially familiar; this, too, may be distracting.

Private Agenda.   Ideas, plans, and any general thoughts in your mind other than what the speaker is telling you distract from your paying careful attention to all that the patient says both denotatively and connotatively. If you are too busy thinking about your own ideas, plans, and, perhaps, responses to the person to pay attention to what he or she is saying, you are not getting all the value you can from listening.

Stereotypes.   Having fixed assumptions and expectations of people because of the general group in which they belong (i.e., in terms of race, religion, age, sex, education, vocation, etc.) can cause you to listen only for those responses which seem to you to fit the stereotypes you have of that group; you may be "mentally deaf" to information that does not fit your idea of that person. For example, a young female dental auxiliary may perceive an older male patient to be sexist and expect him to behave as such, thereby not attending to some information important to a dental history.

Selective Listening.   Closely related to the previous two listening distractions is listening only for selected information, taking words and meanings out of their intended encoded context. Intermittent listening, caused by any of the other distractions listed, can result in selective listening. Hearing only what you expect to hear, what you want to hear, or what you have time to hear during your own silent planning is a form of discrimination in listening which filters out the total message being sent to you. You have prejudged what is worth listening to and what is unimportant.

Patient's Speech Habits.   *How* a speaker talks, rather than what is said, can be distracting if he or she has vocal traits that are extremely different from those you are used to hearing. Nasal pitch, regional dialects, unfamiliar pronunciation, awkward articulation, and other vocal aspects of speech can cause listening distractions if they cause you to become judgmental about them or to become overly curious or concerned about them.

Role Expectations.   Specifically in dental practice, the ways in which you perceive your role as either a dental assistant or a dental hygienist and how you perceive the role of the people labeled "patients" can affect the manner in which you listen to them. If you feel that in the dental operatory you are powerful and they are weak, an assertive, unintimidated patient may "break role" and catch you off-guard so that you do not listen carefully to the verbal message. Likewise, if a patient elaborates in extended detail to answers which you have predetermined need only a short response, and if your authority role expectation is strong, you might cut off the patient's answer. You could do this silently in your own mind and start thinking of something else or you could verbally or nonverbally interrupt the patient. Complete listening is thus impaired because you may otherwise miss valuable feedback which you did not expect.

DEFENSIVENESS AND SILENT ARGUING.   If a speaker is judgmental or critical of a listener, there is a temptation on the part of the listener to become defensive and react to the speaker. The reaction can be either verbal or nonverbal. A verbal reaction might be, "No! You're wrong." A nonverbal reaction might be reflected in a facial expression while the listener silently begins to build up a mental argument against what the speaker has said. Both of these related responses are listening problems because they cause the listener to become so emotionally and personally involved that he/she may not be able to remain at a "professional distance" in an objective way with the speaker. This is true especially in professional relationships with persons who have had less education and experience in a particular field. If a dental patient becomes knowledgeable about some phase of preventive dental care and begins explaining this to a dental professional, the professional may feel that the patient does not have the authority to speak and may begin to turn off the listening ear, silently arguing until the moment is open for a quick retort. When silent arguing begins, active listening stops.

IMPATIENCE.   This is a common listening problem caused by a busy agenda and an eagerness to get on with business. Impatience brings with it the twin problem of having a private agenda. But just wanting to get on with business or on to the next item on a schedule can cause a listener to miss a total message. The listener loses eye contact with the speaker and begins mentally and physically to do something else.

Guidelines for Good Listening

There are ways in which you can be a better listener. Here are a few basic rules which would help to keep the above problems from interfering with your listening:

1. Maintain eye contact with the speaker.
2. Listen empathetically by trying to put yourself in the place of the speaker, understanding the dialogue from his or her point of view.
3. Keep an open mind, not allowing your own assumptions, expectations, value judgments, stereotypes, or personal preferences to filter what the speaker is saying.

4. Listen to every word.
5. Avoid silent debating or private agenda planning.
6. Distinguish between connotative and denotative language.
7. Accept the speaker's feelings, whether you agree with them or not.
8. Observe how a person speaks, noting what the vocal varieties might mean while avoiding any judgment about annoying speech habits that would interfere with your listening.
9. Observe nonverbal–nonvocal communication, noting behavior that helps you understand the speaker's words, avoiding any value judgment about such behavior.
10. Keep mental or written notes about messages you need to have clarified, trying to ask for a clarification at the earliest pause so as not to allow your questions to be on your mind while the speaker continues talking.

It should help you to go over this brief list of listening guidelines several times so that when you do begin an interview they will be second nature to you.

EVALUATING PATIENTS' RESPONSES

Patient responses vary, just as the human conditions change for every individual. The same interview question you ask of one person may elicit a different response from the next person. Because people are different, responses are different and are seldom predictable. And while behavioral modification psychology does offer suggestions to produce predictable behavior, communication for interviewing is somewhat different than communication for behavioral change. There are some common types of responses, however, found frequently in dental settings. Let us look at the most common of these, and comment on ways in which you can deal with them.

   1. *I like you; I feel comfortable being here, and I choose to be responsible for my preventive dental care.* This response is positive toward you, the environment, and the experience of dental care. Your best way of dealing with this type of response is to reinforce the patient's positive attitudes with appreciation, recognition of good dental care, and a positive attitude.
   2. *I like you; I don't like being here; yet I need to be here.* This response is positive toward you, negative toward the immediate situation, but positive toward dental care. The long-range payoff of preventive dental care overcomes the short-term discomfort. This response indicates some intellectual ability by the patient to discipline his or her decisions. You can best deal with logic and long-term goals, together with your own strong role credibility, in this case. Reasoning rather than emotion will work best here.

3. *I have been coming here for twenty years as I have today for my checkup and cleaning and polishing, but I don't feel comfortable with you.* Although this response indicates that the patient has positive feelings about dentistry and his or her own role in preventive dental care, he or she has negative feelings about you. If you have not seen this patient previously, you can begin to develop your own credibility in the professional way in which you work and with a friendly attitude toward the patient; positive feedback to the patient likely will elicit positive adjustments in the patient's attitude and communication. If the patient has been with you previously, you might try to paraphrase what has been said, then ask why the patient feels this way toward you. Being defensive will only make matters worse. Showing that your work is at a professional level may solve the problem.

4. *You seem to be O.K.; but I'm really scared about being here and afraid of what might happen; I always hate coming to the dental office.* Here, you are the only element in the scene which elicits a positive response and the burden for improving matters falls on your shoulders. Talking to the patient about other interests and allowing him or her to talk as much as possible, reassuring the patient about the care and attention given by the dentist, and other positive behavior on your part should help. If time allows, asking open-ended questions about why the patient feels this way might help reduce the problem.

5. *I like you; this is a nice place to be; but I'm not looking forward to seeing the dentist.* The dentist means trouble to this person but you are seen to be on the patient's side. You can serve as a bridge between patient and dentist. Positive statements about the dentist and the dentist's skills may help. Allow the patient the freedom to express his or her feelings, however, and accept these feelings for what they are.

6. *I don't like you; I hate being here now; and I probably won't cooperate with you.* Hostility toward you, the place, and the experience describes this response. Reasoning may not work well with an emotional response. However, being defensive will only reinforce the hostility. You can deal with this response by maintaining a positive attitude in a professional manner toward the patient, acknowledging the patient's feelings, verbally, and allowing him or her to see that you are not judging the patient's feelings. Asking factual questions and keeping the conversation on a logical basis will steer it away from the emotion-laden words which could reinforce the hostility. Objectivity is important here.

7. *Why do I have to be here? I hate coming here. Who are you?* There is hostility toward the situation and indifference about you; you are just another object, part of the total scenery. You could catch flack, too, or you could become a positive element in the person's perception of the preventive dental-care experience. When the patient has no particular feelings about you, you have the opportunity to set the conditions by which the patient *will*

have expectations of you. You could choose to answer the first question in an educational way; the patient may not listen, however. You could ask why the patient hates coming here, although this may be a trap into which you fall—getting into a no-win debate which leads to a more difficult work situation. Developing rapport between the patient and yourself and talking about things the patient does like may help deal with this response.

8. *Well, here I am again (smiles); do whatever needs to be done.* This is either a very passive response or one of resignation bordering on despair. Although it may appear to be cooperative, it is not, because there is no expression of the patient's willingness to be an active participant in his or her own preventive dental care. You can deal with this by talking with the patient in a nonauthoritarian way, helping that person to make some decisions based on his or her own knowledge and self-interest. Such patients tend to place dental professionals on an authoritarian pedestal and succumb. Giving patients some authority over themselves might help.

9. *Silence.* This response could indicate fear, passive hostility, or boredom. It may be an extremely closed response, connotating a tight defense in what is perceived as a threatening, new, or strange environment. One way to deal with this is to try to talk with the patient and ask a few open-ended questions about his or her general interests. One CDA has discovered that talking about rock music stars with teenage patients is often an ice-breaker. However, this nonverbal response of silence is a message and it may simply be saying, "I don't want to talk; just clean and polish my teeth and get it over with." In such a case, this may be all you need to do. You need not impose your own social personality on the patient who chooses to be closed. One patient we know, who is generally silent, is a busy business executive who looks forward to a chance to relax without decisions to make. He likes going to both the barber and the dentist because he can sit down, close his eyes, and be away from his daily pressures; he goes into a near-meditative state when in both a dental chair and a barber's chair. Knowing your patient's needs may help you deal with their silence.

In each of the above responses there are three elements to look for: the patient's attitude toward you, the patient's attitude toward the immediate situation, and the patient's attitude toward his or her own preventive dental-care responsibilites. Recognizing which of these is positive, which neutral, and which negative will help you deal with patients' responses when you encounter them.

SUMMARY

A dental auxiliary interviews a patient to obtain information that will be helpful to the delivery of preventive dental care. There are ten types of techniques that are the key to good interviewing: open-ended questions, closed questions, repetition, interpretive or clarifying responses, probing responses, leading questions or statements, the use of paraphrasing, nonverbal encouragement, summarizing, and closure. Closely related to what you *say* in a dental interview is the *listening* that you do. There are nine listening problems that may occur in a dental setting: noises, patient behavior and appearance, paying attention to one's private agenda, being distracted by stereotypes, selective listening, attending to speech habits rather than content, being distracted by role expectations, defensiveness and silent arguing, and impatience. The listener, can correct problems that interfere with good listening techniques by using the following basic rules: maintain eye contact, listen empathetically, keep an open mind, listen to every word, avoid silent debating, distinguish between connotative and denotative language, accept the speaker's feelings, observe how a person speaks, observe nonverbal–nonvocal communication behaviors, keep mental and written notes. Possible patient responses during a dental interview include (1) I like you, feel comfortable being here, and choose to accept responsibility for my own dental health; (2) I like you, but don't like being here; (3) I don't feel comfortable with you, but I don't mind being here because I'm used to coming to this office; (4) You seem O.K. but I am really scared about being here; (5) I like you and feel comfortable here, but I am not looking forward to seeing the dentist; (6) I don't like you and I probably will not cooperate; (7) I hate coming here—who are you?; (8) Here I am again—do whatever you have to do; (9) Silence. Interviewing in the dental office incorporates all forms of communication including vocal, verbal, written, and nonverbal–nonvocal.

CHAPTER ACTIVITIES

1. Write an example of, or describe, each of the following types of interview technique:
   a. Open-ended question
   b. Closed question
   c. Repetition
   d. Interpretative or clarifying response
   e. Leading question
2. Paraphrase this sentence: "Well, you know how it is; I'm old and, you know, don't have all my teeth; but, I take care of 'em as good as I can—without seeing to well, you know—and I'm not rich enough to go buy all that fancy toothpaste and floss and stuff like that."
3. List the nine listening problems described in this chapter.
4. What are two observations about a patient's communication which you can make as a listener?
5. If a patient tells you that she hates being in a dental office and finds the

whole experience horrible, yet she likes you as a person, what could you say to her before dental work actually begins?

SUGGESTED REFERENCES

Alfred Benjamin, *The Helping Interview*, 2nd ed. (Boston: Houghton Mifflin, 1974).

Lewis Bernstein, Rosalyn Bernstein, and Richard Dana, *Interviewing: A Guide for Health Professionals* (New York: Appleton-Century-Crofts, 1974).

Lawrence M. Bramer, *The Helping Relationship Process and Skills* (Englewood Cliffs, N.J.: Prentice-Hall, 1973).

Allen J. Enelow and Scott N. Swisher, *Interviewing and Patient Care*, 2nd ed. (New York: Oxford University Press, 1979).

Raymond S. Ross, *Speech Communication*, 5th ed. (Englewood Cliffs, N.J.: Prentice-Hall, 1980).

Education, Motivation, and Persuasion

8

What does the phrase "preventive dental care" mean to you? If you are a member of a dental team which believes in preventive dentistry, what does this mean about your role with patients? Generally, *preventive* dental care implies that patients care enough about their teeth and gums to take proper care of them. It also implies that you and the other dental professionals on the team care about preventing oral/dental diseases. This, in turn, means that the patient is expected to do something to prevent problems. But how do the patients know what to do? Can you assume that they learn at home or in school as they grow from infancy into adulthood? And, if they have the knowledge and information, can you assume that they will be motivated to practice what they know? If not, is there anything you as a dental auxiliary can do to influence a change in their attitude and behavior? Experience has shown us that learning, motivating, and persuasion all need to occur and to be reinforced throughout life for dental patients—and the role of the dental auxiliary may well be one of educator, motivator, and persuader.

Dental hygienists work directly with patients for the care of their teeth. Dental assistants work with dentists who practice preventive dentistry; together, they can all develop educational, motivational, and persuasive approaches with patients.

This chapter treats education, motivation, and persuasion separately; but we realize that all are interrelated in actual application in preventive dentistry. All three—learning, motivating, and persuading—rely upon communication. And all three generally result in change.

LEARNING THEORIES

Definition of Learning

What can be said about learning? Here are some basic observations. Learning is the process of acquiring new knowledge and/or skills. It arises out of a need to cope with some aspect of life—mental, physical, or social. It involves change because once we have learned something new we are, to some degree, different. Usually, learning comes about as a result of a relationship between two or more people or between one person and something else in the natural or technological world. Reading a book is a relationship between the reader and the author, but it is also a relationship between the reader and the printed page. In both cases, we learn to relate our needs to the source of answers. Also, learning is selective. We do not have time to learn everything there is to know or to do everything there is to do. We choose what we should learn, often based on our needs to cope. Finally, learning is grounded in experience. We learn through experience and we test our learning by experience.

There are many theories of learning. We are concerned with those which apply to the circumstances in which dental hygienists work, and in which dental assistants and dentists work together as a team.

Satisfying Needs

One learning theory says that learning occurs when a person has a need that can be satisfied by acquiring new information and/or new skills. It is the relationship between the need and that which satisfies the need which is learned. That is, we learn how to satisfy needs. If bridging the gap between need and satisfaction requires knowledge, we try to acquire the knowledge. If it requires a new skill, we try to learn the skill. A patient may recognize that he is consistently told by a hygienist that he develops an unacceptable amount of plaque on his teeth every six months. The patient decides that he needs to learn a better way to clean his teeth. The dental hygienist gives him information and shows him a new technique for controlling the problem. The patient's needs become satisfied. He learns a relationship between a skill and the need for cleaner teeth. He also has learned another relationship—namely, that a dental hygienist can help provide information and skills that are conducive to preventive dental care. If he wants more information, he knows where to go. It is similar to learning how to read a map.

This learning theory includes not only knowledge and skills but also values and subjective meaning. It is, therefore, "good" to have clean teeth and healthy gums. To hold this value for oneself will allow one to determine what is necessary to learn. A person determines what is of value and importance and then proceeds to try to learn these things.

Persons associated with this theory of learning are Edward C. Tolman, who developed concepts dealing with both psychological and physiological needs, and Kurt Lewin, who related meaning and values to motivation.[1]

According to this theory, much of the learning that occurs is necessarily motivated by the patient. The dental professional might take some initiative in providing information that would make a patient aware of a need, but it would be the patient's own values which would motivate him or her to learn a relationship (knowledge or skill) that would satisfy that need. Then, the dental professional would assist in providing information. Communication is a process of information sharing, and thereby makes learning possible. The purpose is to inform, but not to persuade or motivate. Motivation precedes learning as a result of a patient's own values and choices.

Behavior Management

A second learning theory has developed from the work of B. F. Skinner. This theory was demonstrated in the 1930s when Skinner showed that giving positive rewards to laboratory animals reinforced the specific kind of behavior they were being taught. Likewise, negative responses were given animals for inappropriate behavior. Today, teaching machines, programmed learning, and behavioral modification have evolved from Skinner's theory of "operant conditioning."[2]

The theory of learning by conditioning deals with those lessons which are purposefully and intentionally taught. They do not deal with what are called "elicited responses" such as shivering in response to cold or blinking as a response to sudden bright light. Rather, it deals with specific *actions* of the subject based on learned experiences. It is the difference between a knee jerk in response to a mild tap during a physical exam, and the intentional knee action of a football player kicking a field goal. The latter is learned and reinforced by positive rewards—more points on the scoreboard.

This theory is popular among classroom teachers and parents, and is often used to manage children's behavior in socially acceptable ways. One factor that is important to the success of this form of learning is frequent and consistent reinforcement. This is the one major drawback for this theory as applied to the work of a dental professional because of the infrequency of patient-professional contacts. It would be very difficult to give positive rewards to a patient of any age who you do not see more than once every six months. In the meantime, many other forms of behavior can go unmanaged. For example, you can tell a patient how well he or she is doing at flossing, using all the facial and verbal messages at your command to give a positive "reward" to that person. But to receive this reinforcement information only twice a year does not give a patient the frequency that may be necessary to stimulate him or her to learn and to change behavior.

However, the behavioral changes can be conditioned by others who do see the patient daily, such as school teachers, and parents, and even other members of the person's peer group. So a dental hygienist may be able to chart a course for a parent in how to reward a child when the desired technique is performed by the child. One way to do this, for example, is for the parent to give the child something the child values each time the desired behavior is followed. Candy would not be appropriate for dental care (although it *is* used frequently by parents and teachers as a reward). Verbal recognition might be useful—openly acknowledging that the child has done the correct procedure each time he or she brushes and flosses. Whatever reward the parent or teacher perceive as a positive or negative response will be what ultimately functions as the reward.

Operant conditioning generally does not deal with motives or values in that it does not try to teach internal philosophies or rationale. It is concerned with consequences of behavior, the observable actions of a person. It is left to the individual to develop his or her own values regarding the behavior.

Although we do not believe that operant conditioning is practical for dental professionals working with patients on an infrequent and irregular basis, we do believe that it is useful for parents and teachers to use with children and with adult patients to apply themselves in a kind of self-disciplined behavior management program. Its advantage is that it is selective—that is, it works best when applied to a specific behavior one wishes to learn (change). In this case, a specific behavior might be "to substitute nonsweetened snacks for sugar candy," or "to floss each time you brush." Conditioned learning does seem to have direct application to preventive dental care, but more on the part of the patient than on the part of the dental professional. Your task as a dental auxiliary may be, over the long term, to show the positive relationship between patient behavior and improved dental hygiene.

Competency

A third learning theory postulates that the development of competency is the essence of education. It is learning to do something new, to be aware of something new, or to understand something new. Whereas the two previous theories deal with learning as the result of some previous stimulus or need-satisfying activity, this theory, in contrast, centers on the value of things learned as they relate to the *later* achievement of a desired behavior. By learning some skill prior to the time we need to use the skill, and not because we will be rewarded for doing it, we can even make some tentative prediction about the effectiveness of what we learn. What is sought in such learning is not a specific skill, as one might learn through operant conditioning, but an ability to sort out elements in any situation which one needs for a useful purpose. For example, as we go through a supermarket, how do we know *what* to select out of all the varieties of produce available? How do we know *how* to select what we want? If we have learned in advance what to look for and how to test its suitability, then it can be predicted that the salad we will make when we get home will be what we wanted before we walked into the supermarket. Robert Gagné has shown that if we can become familiar with a situation before having to act in that situation, we will learn how to act more quickly when the actual situation arises.[3] Joseph Scandura goes a step further and shows that one does not even need to understand the nature of a problem in order to deal with it.[4] If one has developed competent problem-solving skills, he or she can apply those skills in most situations effectively without needing to understand the problem in great depth. Scandura's study seems to indicate that it is not massive amounts of information and analyses that we need in order to solve problems; rather, it is the skill of problem solving which we need first. As this applies to learning, we would, therefore, teach people skills before they need them. The best way, then, to be prepared is through advance simulations and "rehearsing" of various skills, either mentally or experimentially.

This theory is applicable to a situation in which a dental hygienist, for example, is teaching a person how to use a toothbrush or how to floss in order to prevent possible future dental problems. Using visual aids such as charts, oversized brush, and teeth models, or even using yourself as a model, you can instruct a patient in the proper brushing motions. Using a mirror so that the patients can see themselves, you can let them see how they are doing while they are in the operatory. Then, with this skill once begun, the patient can go home and repeat the correct process. This learning leads to competency. The patient does not need to know all the reasons why the way you teach is best in preventive dental care. Nor does the patient, according to Scandura's theory, need to know all the relevant information about dental development and decay. *You* may need to know it, but the patient probably does not in order to practice preventive dental care. This does not mean that information is hidden or denied the patient. It simply means that learning a skill with competency does not first require learning all the information related to the problem.

Fear Reduction

A fourth learning theory, developed by O.H. Mowrer and others, emphasizes the role of anxiety or acquired fear in what we learn. Whatever will reduce anxiety or fear is what is learned and maintained. An aspect of this theory which may be directly relevant to dental professionals is the suggestion by Mowrer than when even a neutral stimulus, one which in itself evokes no fear,

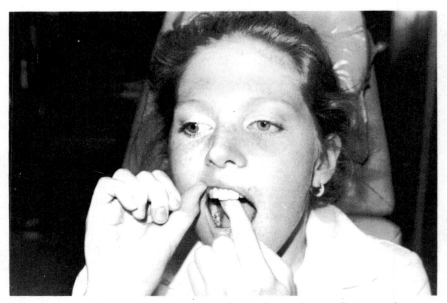

Figure 8–1. Here the patient looks in the mirror to learn effective flossing techniques. Having the patient floss in the dental office helps to reinforce the skill so the patient can go home and repeat the techniques accurately.

is accidentally presented at the same time as a painful stimulus, a person will associate even the neutral stimulus with pain. A dental patient could learn to be afraid of dental-care situations by associating the pain of one event with something as innocent as the white uniform worn by dental assistants at the time of the next visit. The anxiety could be stimulated because of a past association. Mowrer differentiates between emotional responses and physiological responses; it is the emotional responses, such as fear, that are learned, while physiological responses are voluntary and mostly under control of the central nervous system.[5]

Conclusions about Learning Theories

Each of the four theories of learning briefly outlined above express a particular viewpoint concerning the nature of learning. Each is supported by careful study and each claims a degree of validity. What we in the dental health field need to know is *what works.* From this perspective, it might be safe to say that no one theory is applicable to every learning situation. As is true of all communication situations, learning is influenced by the goals, objectives, persons involved, the purpose of the occasion, the amount of time available, and other variables. Individually, people learn in different ways, governed by the existing conditions.

In a study done by one of the authors, in which a personalized system of instruction (PSI) was used, students were allowed to study material at their own rate, with emphasis placed on mastery of subject matter rather than on academic grades. In a control group, another class was taught by a lecture method, with everyone having to go at the same pace and being rewarded by grades in comparison with everyone else. The results of the study showed not that one system was better than another for everyone, but that some students developed competency in a self-paced approach and some did not. Likewise, some excelled in a traditional lecture–discussion format and some did not. The conclusions led to speculation that, among other things, it was not the system but the individual student's own way of learning which affected the competency.

Some teachers are very effective using a lecture monologue approach, others achieve results by using a dialogue method, and others employ experiential learning methods. People learn in different ways, and teachers teach effectively in different ways.

TWO LEARNING APPROACHES

Taking whichever theory applies to your situation, you can apply it to various teaching approaches. Basically, there are two approaches that might be used by a dental professional with a patient. One we can call the *deductive* approach; the other is the *inductive* approach.

The Deductive Approach

The deductive method is one in which the teacher (dental hygienist, dentist, etc.) tells the student (patient) what he or she needs to know or how to perform a particular skill. This method is quick and relies on clarity of verbal communication. It also requires that the student (patient) be a good listener and be able to understand, accept, and internalize what is being said. It requires some degree of dialogue, as outlined in Chapter 1, where we noted that communication only finally occurs after the message goes through a seven-stage process of development. Basically, this approach is used for giving instructions and teaching basic skills by showing the receiver various charts, pictures, and models. All the speech skills described in Chapter 5 come into play here. In the short amount of time a patient is with you in the operation, this may be the method you would choose under most routine, regular teaching situations—for example, telling a child which foods are good for the health of his or her teeth and which are harmful.

The Inductive Approach

The inductive method starts with the student (patient). The student *discovers* the truth about something by following a system you, the teacher, devise. With this method there is more active participation in learning on the student's part. The teacher guides the process and checks the progress. *Learning by experience* might be the best way to describe this.

An example of this form of teaching/learning is illustrated in Figure 8–2, in which a dental hygienist is shown (a) brushing the patient's teeth; the patient holds a mirror so she can see the process; and then (b) the patient is asked to try brushing in different ways. Once the teacher (hygienist) observes how the patient manipulates the brush, she can comment on the effectiveness of this process with the patient (student). An even better example of this "discovery" learning method is the use of disclosing solution on the teeth to help a patient learn eventually which methods of cleaning and flossing will be most effective. This procedure exemplifies operant conditioning, the reward being stain-free teeth after practicing the most effective brushing/flossing technique. However, in some situations it might not be preferable to let a patient, especially a child, learn by the trial and error, or discovery, method what foods are best for healthy teeth. In this case the hygienist's specific teaching is best.

Frank Wentz, describing the importance of establishing the educational needs of patients, refers to a study by A. A. Ariando in which the patient's understanding of the role of bacteria in the disease process is shown to positively reinforce his or her motivation to use unwaxed floss.[6]

To achieve the goal of preventive dental care, the theory of learning and the teaching method would be determined primarily, therefore, by the situation and the objectives, not by determining which theory is "best" or "most effective." Effectiveness is determined by the individual situation. Knowing when to apply each theory and when to use each method requires a degree of flexibility, as does any effective communication behavior.

MOTIVATION

Learning and motivation usually go hand in hand. Most of the learning theories developed by psychologists and educators include motivation within their theory. (For example, Skinner's experiment with operant conditioning used laboratory animals that were hungry, presumably so they would be motivated to learn to trigger the lever which would mechanically reward them with food pellets.) *Motivation*, simply put, is what compels an individual, internally, to act.

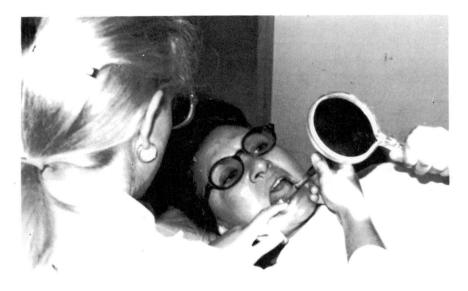

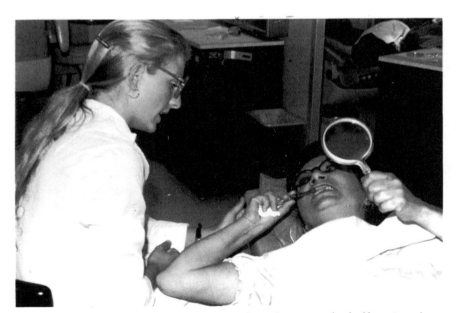

Figure 8–2 (a and b). These photos illustrate the inductive method of learning. A patient learns by doing.

Hierarchy of Needs

Abraham Maslow, in developing his well-known hierarchy of human needs, pointed to different levels of human need which motivate individuals to strive for different goals and objectives throughout life. Advertisers often use this hierarchy to develop advertising which they hope will motivate people first to pay attention to the message and second to purchase the product. If physiological needs (such as for sex, food, shelter) are basic to all humans, an advertiser might use words, pictures, and colors that relate to these needs, thereby capturing the viewer's attention and, perhaps, motivating purchase of the product. Knowing at what need level an individual is operating at any given moment is the key to using such an approach. In dental practice, the need of a patient might be for safety, if pain is associated with dental care; or for a sense of belonging, if the patient wants teeth that are pleasing to look at and will thereby help in achievement of social acceptability. Even though some toothpaste advertisements attempt to relate love and belonging needs to white teeth, we believe that such an appeal misleads an individual into a false understanding of what makes a relationship meaningful. However, self-esteem may well be a valid need level at which a message could be directed, especially if one believes that care of one's physical self—including oral hygiene—is a part of one's total well-being. This is an example of the learning theory in which personal values relate to a person's motivation; if you value your physical health and if taking care of your physical condition contributes to feeling good about yourself, you will be motivated to learn how to care for your teeth. Likewise, if a person's teeth were in such bad condition that pain hindered eating, it would make sense to make use of the basic physiological need to avoid pain. Maslow's hierarchy of needs may well have an application to understanding motivation of dental patients. Figure 8–3 illustrates Maslow's hierarchy of needs.

Fear as a Motivator

There are other ways of looking at motivation. One classic study in the dental health field was done by I. L. Janis and H. Feshbach in 1953. They studied the importance of fear as a motivation for getting people to care for their teeth.[7] Their study used three different messages with three levels of fear appeal. Their fear levels were varied by changes in the type of visual aids used to illustrate a lecture. They wanted to determine the effects of strong, moderate, and minimal fear appeals on the way in which the audience followed suggested dental hygiene practices.

The minimal fear visual aids used X-rays and drawings to illustrate cavities, and photographs to show healthy teeth. Moderate appeal visual aids were photographs of mild cases of tooth decay and oral diseases. Strong fear appeal visual aids used photographic slides to show realistic cases of ad-

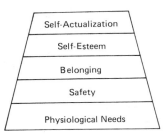

Figure 8-3. Maslow's hierarchy of needs. (Data (for diagram) based on Hierarchy of Needs in "A Theory of Human Motivation" in *Motivation and Personality*, Second Edition by Abraham H. Maslow. Copyright © 1970 by Abraham H. Maslow. Reprinted by permission of Harper & Row, Publishers, Inc.)

vanced tooth decay and oral diseases, and included the words "This can happen to you." A control group was given a lecture on the human eye. The four groups—those having been exposed to one of the three fear appeal levels and the control group—were given questionnaires one week before and one week after the lectures asking specific questions about their personal dental care. Results showed that more of those who received the *moderate* fear appeal followed the recommendations in the lecture. The dental-care habits of those who were exposed to the strong fear appeal changed the least. This indicates that strong fear used as a motive to follow prescribed dental hygiene practices is not necessarily effective.

Attitude and Behavior Change

One problem connected with using motivation to get people to learn concerns the difference between *attitude change* and *behavioral change*. If you can change a person's attitude about preventive dental care, can you be assured that he or she will change actual behavior? And, if you do change it (or if they change it themselves) over the short term, how long will the behavioral change last? Parents, for example, may be convinced that flossing should accompany brushing, and even insist that their children follow a regular practice of flossing after brushing. But the parents may not themselves practice what they believe is important for the children. Leon Festinger, a psychologist interested in the relationship between attitude change and behavior change, noted that in the Janis and Feshbach study of fear appeals, the persons in the study had reported an inverse relationship between attitude change and behavior change.[8]

On the other side of the coin, some studies of behavior change indicate a "sleeper effect"—i.e., a change of behavior after an idea has had time to "germinate" in the mind of the person who has been sent a persuasive message.

GROUP CONSENSUS.   One of the more helpful studies of how people change attitudes *and* behavior was done by Kurt Lewin during World War II, when the U.S. Department of Agriculture was interested in developing a change in food habits in the United States. The results of this study have since given credence to the Group Dynamics movement in this country. The study used two teaching methods to present information about nutrition, economics, and methods of preparing unpopular meat cuts. One group of housewives received a lecture, accompanied by printed handouts of recipes. A second group was given some initial information but encouraged to discuss the information in small groups. The food preparation and home economics information was made available only as group members felt the need for such information. A followup by the same researcher showed that while only 3 percent of the women in the lecture group actually followed up on the suggestions, 32 percent of those in the discussion–decision-making group had served at least one of the meat suggestions.[9] One conclusion from this study which might be relevant to dental hygiene and preventive dental care was that *group consensus was an important motivating factor.* In other words, it was not the authority of a lecturer which effected change, but the decision made by the individuals themselves, supported by others who made the same decision.

This approach to motivation may not seem useful outside a group, a situation in which a dental professional rarely works. Most dental care is done on a one-on-one basis through interpersonal communication. However, the view that *an individual will be more likely to be motivated if he or she is an active part of the decision to change* has support on the interpersonal level as well as on the group level.

IMPORTANCE OF EMPATHY.   Samuel F. Dworkin, after comparing psychoanalytic and behavioristic methods of attitude change, concluded that it is the empathy of the dental professional toward the patient that is most helpful.[10] This coincides with a conclusion reached by Carl Rogers, who studied the effectiveness of professional counselors and psychologists using different therapeutic and analytical methods. His conclusion was that no matter what helping technique was used, the patients who believed that they were helped most were those who felt that their professional helper was most *empathetic* toward them.[11]

A dental hygienist, assistant, or dentist who shows sincere concern about the patient, listens to feedback with understanding, and acknowledges the patient's own concern (including fear and anxiety) without being judgmentally critical, will have a good chance to help the patient develop a long-term behavior change toward preventive dental care.

Knowing how a patient perceives the dental professional (dentist, hygienist, or assistant) is important not only to your understanding of how to motivate a patient. It is just as important to understand why a patient may or may not be motivated to seek preventive dental care at all. In a study done with 430 employees of the same company, which had a company-paid dental-care plan, S. Stephan Kegeles found that three psychological factors were potential barriers to seeking preventive dental care: (1) fear of pain, (2) anxiety about what might happen, and (3) negative perception of the dentist.[12] In our chapter on perception, you may recall, we discussed the importance of perception in communication, and mentioned the importance of dental auxiliaries in helping patients acknowledge and overcome their negative perception of the dentist. This element was missing from Kegeles' study. However, he did discuss the factors that were influential in leading people to have a positive attitude toward seeking dental care. Among these were (1) a belief that one is susceptible to dental disease, (2) a belief that dental treatment is beneficial, (3) an esthetic concern for one's teeth, (4) a lack of anxiety about dental treatment, (5) lack of fear of pain, and (6) a positive appraisal of the dentist.[13] We believe that knowing these factors that contribute to motivating people to seek dental health is helpful to the dental auxiliary.

At the beginning of this chapter, we said that learning, motivation, and persuasion were interrelated. It is difficult to discuss aspects of any one of these communication activities without discussing the other two. Indeed, motivation and persuasion may seem to be synonymous to you. So, now that we have investivated learning and motivation as they may relate to your work as a dental auxiliary, we shall discuss persuasion as an integral part of your work with people who seek dental care.

COMMUNICATION EXERCISE 8-1

Consider the things that motivate you in your daily life. Below is a list of a limited number of factors that motivate individuals. Check the space that is applicable to you for each factor. Then add additional factors that affect you in your daily living.

	Always	Most of the Time	Occasionally	Never
1. Positive comments				
2. Negative comments				
3. Feeling hurt				
4. Being mad				
5. Feeling empathetic				
6. Believing in				
7. Hunger				
8. Group pressure and consensus				
9. Time				
10. Fear				
11. Pain				
12. Disapointment				

(continued)

COMMUNICATION EXERCISE 8-1 *(Contd)*

	Always	Most of the Time	Occasionally	Never
14. Success				
15. Failure				
16.				
17.				
18.				
19.				
20.				

PERSUASION

For our purposes we differentiate between learning, motivation, and persuasion by definitions which apply to your work in preventive dental care. Whereas *learning* is defined as the acquisition of knowledge or a skill, and *motivation* is defined as that which internally compels an individual to act, *persuasion* is defined here in terms of *external influence*. Learning depends on the motivation within a person but may be prompted by outside persuasion. Or, to put it another way, a dental auxiliary may, through persuasion, motivate a patient to learn something that will change that person's attitude and/or behavior.

     The emphasis in this final part of the chapter, then, is on your influence on persons seeking preventive dental care. Much of your part in persuasion has already been covered in Part I and Part II of this book. Roles, perceptions, and communication choices all combine now in your effort to teach, motivate, and persuade.

Guideline to Becoming Persuasive

If you wish to influence another person so that he or she will be motivated to learn (change), there are some basic steps which we recommend you follow.

     1. *Be aware of your own attitudes about yourself and about the person you wish to persuade.* (We discussed this earlier in the sections on self-concept and roles.) Being honest about such attitudes will, to some degree, affect your manner of verbal and nonverbal communication. This in itself determines the interpersonal environment in which the patient becomes either receptive or defensive regarding your attempts to persuade him or her to change dental habits or undertake new ones.

2. Be knowledgeable about what it is you wish to communicate through your influence. Know what you are talking about. This knowledge comes from other teachers, textbooks, simulated learning, and actual clinical experience. Presumably, a dental auxiliary who becomes either a Certified Dental Assistant or a Registered Dental Hygienist does have satisfactory knowledge of the subject of preventive dental care.

3. *Know your purpose.* Your purpose is directly related to the overall goal of preventive dental care. A purpose, in terms of influence, is a specific, observable, clearly stated objective the results of which you will be able to observe if the patient does indeed learn and become motivated to follow your suggestions. For example, you might state your purpose like this: "I want to persuade the patient to follow a regular, twice-daily routine of brushing and flossing."

4. *Analyze the needs and desires of the patient.* Try to identify those needs which the patient can identify. Also, identify the needs which the patient may not be able to describe. Try to identify the patient's beliefs and values as they relate to preventive dental care. These will have to do with his or her own motives for seeking dental care. For example, does the patient value the esthetic value of attractive teeth and gums? By such analysis you will be able to enter into a meaningful dialogue with the patient, even in a brief period of time, in order to begin to get him or her involved in making decisions about personal oral hygiene goals.

Persuasive Communication

Once you have established these four preliminary steps, you can follow five additional steps that will help you become a persuasive communicator.[14]

1. *Get the attention of your listener.* We recommend that you develop attention in an empathetic way by showing concern and entering into a dialogue with the patient from the beginning of your encounter in the operatory. If you elicit from the patient himself a perception of you as a credible person (see the section on Trust, Chapter 5), you likely will already have the patient's attention.

2. *Determine the need.* Again, through descriptive statements about the patient's dental condition and through interviewing and active listening techniques (Chapter 7), you can establish what the particular need of the patient is. One need might be for a patient to decrease the amount of snack food containing sugar. During this step, you can describe the problem of eating food with high sugar content and the effects of a high sugar diet. You can, using interviewing techniques, allow the patient to tell you how much soda pop, candy, and sugar-coated cereal he or she consumes each day. As we said in the section on motivation, if a person takes an active part in the

decision-making process, he or she is more likely to be motivated, eventually, by your persuasion. Let the patient say aloud what he or she recognizes as the problem with the diet. This particular step might just as well be labeled the "teaching/learning" step, for it is here that you and the patient exchange information about the problem and arrive at some commonly acknowledged understanding of the need. As was explained in Chapter 1, in the discussion of the seven stages of dialogue, understanding comes *before* acceptance, internalization, or action. The patient should be helped to understand the need.

   3. *Offer a solution to the problem.* This step in interpersonal communication can be provided in a direct descriptive statement, by means of instructions, or by a specific routine for the patient to follow. Or, in a nondirective way, you could ask the patient to state some solutions he or she might think of. Whichever way is used, your own knowledge of acceptable solutions will be a helpful guide to the patient. And, whichever teaching method you use, inductive or deductive, it is best to be very clear and concrete. In the chapter on communication choices we stated that clarity is very important in speech communication. Denotative words may come closer to describing concrete procedures for the patient to follow than connotative words. However, the patient may need some hypothetical illustrations and analogies to understand what you are saying. It is vague to say, "Can you drink less soda pop?" It is clearer to say, for example, "Cutting down from five cans of pop a day to two a day would reduce your sugar diet. Do you think you can do that?" This step offers the patient concrete solutions, whether they be yours or the patient's. It is best to come to a common agreement about the solution if the patient is to be motivated to do what you are teaching.

   4. *Reinforce the suggested solution by using visualization.* Here you can describe what things will be like if the patient does follow the solution. Considering the research by Janis and Feshbach, it might be helpful to show in a *moderate* way what the conditions of the patient's teeth and gums would be like if he or she did not follow your solution. Some visual aid or illustrative verbal examples of the oral effects of a high sugar diet could be used as a mild fear appeal. If the patient can visualize the results, he or she will be able to internalize the message you are sending. Your influence will have progressed a step further.

   5. *Ask for action.* Again, this can be done in a direct appeal such as, "Now that you understand the importance of cutting down on sugar each day, I encourage you to begin today, so that in six months you can show me the results." Or, in a nondirective approach, you can ask the patient to tell you when the new behavior will begin and how many sugar snacks he or she intends to eliminate. You might even ask for substitute snack suggestions which the patient could purchase in place of the sugar-filled snacks. Getting the patient to make a spoken commitment to you may even fit into a self-motivated behavioral management program by the patient! The action step

requests the listener/student/patient to make the desired changes of attitude and behavior.

LEARNING/MOTIVATING/ PERSUADING: A PRACTICAL APPLICATION

Thus far we have described four theories of learning, described some aspects of motivation, and given specific steps for persuasion. Because of the interrelated nature of these topics in actual practice, we conclude this chapter with a practical application of all of these.

Let's assume that you want to see each of your patients practicing a preventive care program which you prescribe. Let's assume, also, that you do not have patients who are from the same background, of the same age, education, or economic status. They are all different. Yet you have a plan which you believe to be a good, simple, effective method for each of them to follow. You want to develop a method of education/motivation/persuasion that will be realistic for the amount of time you have with each patient. Considering the variables of age, education, and experience and the vocabulary that might be adapted to compensate for these variables, what is a good method? There probably is no "best way" for everyone in every situation. Table 8–1 gives an example of one way that applies many of the communication ideas mentioned in this chapter.

SUMMARY

There are a number of learning theories that relate to the circumstances in which dental hygienists work, and in which dental assistants and dentists work together as a team. One theory states that learning occurs when a person has a need that can be satisfied by the acquisition of new information and/or new skills. A second theory, developed from the work of B. F. Skinner, is called operant conditioning. It deals with those things that are purposefully and intentionally taught, and concentrates on the specific actions of the learner based on what is learned. The third theory, especially applicable to the dental situation, is the theory of competency: all learning does not first require knowledge of all the information related to the problem. A fourth theory emphasizes the role of anxiety or acquired fear as the basis for what is learned. There are two teaching approaches which might be used by the dental auxiliary with a patient: deductive and inductive. The deductive method relies on the clarity of verbal communication. The teacher tells the learner what is needed or how to perform the skill. The inductive method, on the

TABLE 8–1. *Examples of Education, Motivation, and Persuasion*

VERBAL COMMUNICATION	NONVERBAL COMMUNICATION	LEARNING/THEORY METHOD	MOTIVATION THEORY	PERSUASION STEP
Preliminary conversation and interview.	Comfortable room. Smile.		Determine need level.	Develop trust.
Describe condition of patient's teeth, gums.	Hand patient mirror.	Need satisfaction.	Individual participation.	Attention.
Ask about eating habits, smoking habits, etc.		Inductive method.		
Ask about patient's desire for improved oral condition, esthetic values.		Values (need satisfaction).	Need.	Need.
Tell patient the consequences of not brushing & flossing correctly.	Show photographs of teeth with mild calculus, inflamed gums.		Mild fear.	
Paraphrase patient's stated wishes (from step 4).		Need satisfaction.		
Ask again about value of esthetics.		Inductive.	Individual participation.	
Identify some "rewards" for patient.		Goals for behavior management.		
Describe your specific methods.	Show chart of correct procedure. Use brush on model.	Need satisfaction.		Solution/satisfaction.

158

Describe how to brush.	Hand patient brush, hold mirror for patient to see own skill.	Competence.	
Tell patient when skill is done correctly.	Smile. Eye contact.	Behavior management.	Fear reduction.
State what foods are good for teeth.	Show wall poster illustrating healthy foods.		
Tell patient that by doing what you have taught and by eating foods with less sugar, oral hygiene will improve.	Show picture of healthy teeth and gums.		
Ask patient to state how often he/she will brush & floss. Ask patient to name sugarless snacks that will substitute for sugar snacks.	Smile. Eye contact.	Competency & need satisfaction.	
Ask when these changes will begin.	Smile when response is given.	Behavior management.	Individual participation.
Tell patient you look forward to seeing the good results at next appointment.	Hand patient brush enscribed with name, in original package, and wallet sized chart of healthy foods and snack suggestions.		

other hand, places responsibility on the learner, who experiences the skill or discovers for himself the needed information. To achieve quality preventive services, the dental auxiliary determines which learning theory and teaching method to use depending on the patient and situation. *Motivation* is defined as what compels an individual, internally, to act. Most of the learning theories discussed included motivation, as an important factor. *Learning* is defined as the acquisition of knowledge or a skill. *Persuasion* consists of the external influences that compel an individual to act. To be influential with patients, the dental auxiliary needs to be aware of her personal attitude about self and patients, to be knowledgeable about the subject, to know the purpose, of the dental care, and to analyze the needs and desires of the patient. The five steps *for effective persuasive communication require the dental auxiliary to* (1) get the attention of the listener, (2) determine the patient's need, (3) offer a solution with a statement about how the need can be satisfied, (4) reinforce the suggested solution, and (5) ask for action.

CHAPTER ACTIVITIES

1. List five different kinds of subjects or skills you have learned in your lifetime. Opposite each, describe in your own words how you have learned the subject or skill. Notice whether each answer describes the same means of learning and determine the differences according to subject or skill.
2. Choose one subject you are studying (or have studied) in school. Describe two different ways in which it might be taught, one inductive, and one deductive.
3. Interview three classmates or associates. Ask what motivates them to brush and floss their teeth. List answers in categories that correspond to the learning or motivation theories described in this chapter.
4. Develop a persuasive message that follows the five-step persuasive communication sequence described in this chapter.

REFERENCES

1. Tolman believes there are six kinds of relationships that are learned. One he calls "cathexes," which is the attachment of a goal to a drive. There are both positive and negative cathexes. See Edward C. Tolman, "There Is More than One Kind of Learning," *Psychological Review*, 56 (1949), 144–55.
2. B. F. Skinner, *The Behavior of Organisms: An Experimental Analysis* (New York: Appleton-Century-Crofts, 1938).
3. Gagné has formulated a "theory of productive learning," in which he describes a hierarchy of subordinate tasks. See Robert Gagné, "The Acquisition of Knowledge," *Psychological Review*, 69 (1962), 355–65.

4. Joseph M. Scandura, "Alogrithm Learning and Problem Solving," *Journal of Experimental Education*, 34 (1966), 1–6.

5. Mowrer believes that habit formation is dependent on feedback and that "positive feedback" is the essence of habit development. See O. H. Mowrer, "Two-Factor Learning Theory Reconsidered with Special Reference to Secondary Reinforcement and the Concept of Habit," *Psychological Review*, 63 (1956), 114–28.

6. A. A. Ariando, "How Frequently Must Patients Carry Out Effective Oral Hygiene Procedures in Order to Maintain Gingival Health?", *Journal of Periodontics*, 42 (May 1971), 309, as cited by Frank M. Wentz, "Patient Motivation: A New Challenge to the Dental Profession for Effective Control of Plaque," *Journal of the American Dental Association*, 85 (October 1972), 889.

7. Described in C. I. Hovland, I. L. Janis, and H. H. Kelley, *Communication and Persuasion* (New Haven: Yale University Press, 1953), pp. 66–73.

8. Leon Festinger, "Behavioral Support for Opinion Change," *Public Opinion Quarterly*, 28 (1964), 404–17.

9. Described in Werner J. Severin and James W. Tankard, Jr., *Communication Theories* (New York: Hastings House, 1979), pp. 147–48.

10. Samuel F. Dworkin, "A Rationale for Obtaining Change in Attitude Behavior of Dental Patients," *Journal of the Tennessee Dental Association*, 53, no. 2 (1973), 152.

11. Carl Rogers, "The Characteristics of a Helping Relationship," in *On Becoming a Person* (Boston: Houghton Mifflin, 1961), pp. 39–57.

12. S. Stephen Kegeles, "Some Motivations for Seeking Preventive Dental Care," *Journal of the American Dental Association*, 67 (July 1963), 90–95.

13. Ibid., p. 90.

14. See Alan H. Monroe and Douglas Ehninger, *Principles of Speech Communication*, 7th ed. (Glenview, Ill.: Scott, Foresman, 1975), pp. 242–45.

BIBLIOGRAPHY

Ariando, A. A., "How Frequently Must Patients Carry Out Effective Oral Hygiene Procedures in Order to Maintain Gingival Health?", *Journal of Periodontics*, 42 (May 1971), 309.

Benjamin, Alfred, *The Helping Interview*. 2nd ed. Boston: Houghton Mifflin, 1974.

Bernstein, Lewis, Bernstein, Rosalyn, and Dana, Richard, *Interviewing: A Guide for Health Professionals*. New York: Appleton-Century-Crofts, 1974.

Bramer, Lawrence M., *The Helping Relationship*. Englewood Cliffs, N.J.: Prentice-Hall, 1973.

Dworkin, Samuel F., "A Rationale for Obtaining Change in Attitude Behavior of Dental Patients," *Journal of the Tennessee Dental Association*, 53, no. 2 (1973), 152.

Enelow, Allen J., and Swisher, Scott, N., *Interviewing and Patient Care*, 2nd ed. New York: Oxford University Press, 1979.

FESTINGER, LEON, "Behavioral Support for Opinion Change," *Public Opinion Quarterly*, 28 (1964), 404–17.

GAGNÉ, ROBERT, "The Acquisition of Knowledge," *Psychological Review*, 69 (1962), 355–65.

HOVLAND, C. I., JANIS, I. L., and KELLEY, H. H., *Communication and Persuasion*. New Haven: Yale University Press, 1953.

KEGELES, STEPHEN, "Some Motivations for Seeking Preventive Dental Care," *Journal of the American Dental Association*, 67 (July 1963), 90–95.

MASLOW, ABRAHAM H., *Motivation and Personality*. New York: Harper & Row, 1954.

MONROE, ALAN H., and EHNINGER, DOUGLAS, *Principles of Speech Communication*. 7th ed., Glenview, Ill.: Scott, Foresman, 1975.

MOWRER, H. O., "Two-Factor Learning Theory Reconsidered with Special Reference to Secondary Reinforcement and the Concept of Habit," *Psychological Review*, 63 (1956), 114–28.

ROGERS, CARL, "The Characteristics of a Helping Relationship," in *On Becoming a Person*. Boston: Houghton Mifflin, 1961.

ROSS, RAYMOND S., *Speech Communication*, 5th ed. Englewood Cliffs, N.J.: Prentice-Hall, 1980.

SCANDURA, JOSEPH, "Alogrithm Learning and Problem Solving," *Journal of Experimental Education*, 34 (1966), 1–6.

SEVERIN, WERNER J., and TANKARD, JAMES W., JR., *Communication Theories*. New York: Hastings House, 1979.

SKINNER, B. F., *The Behavior of Organisms: An Experimental Analysis*. New York: Appleton-Century-Crofts, 1938.

TOLMAN, EDWARD, "There Is More than One Kind of Learning," *Psychological Review*, 56, (1949), 144–45.

WENTZ, FRANK, "Patient Motivation: A New Challenge to the Dental Profession for Effective Control of Plaque," *Journal of the American Dental Association*, 85 (October 1972), 889.

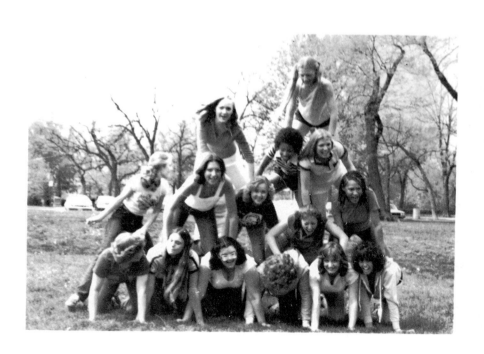

ORGANIZATIONAL COMMUNICATION AND THE DENTAL HEALTH TEAM

IV

When I tell someone what to do, that person is my slave. When I explain the reason for its doing, I have increased his stature. When I let the person plan with me, I have made him a partner.

J. DONALD PHILLIPS*

KEY POINTS

CHAPTER 9
**Definition of a Dental Health
Team**
**Factors Influencing Team Effec-
tiveness**
structured variables
independent or environmental
variables
task-related variables
intermediate variables
dependent variables
**The Needs of People in a Dental
Health Team**
Evolution of a Team
Communication Networks
total system networks
personal networks
cliques
**Building a Successful Dental
Health Team**
guidelines for achieving
cohesiveness

**Dynamics of a Dental Health
Team**
establishing team goals
leadership styles
roles
role ambiguity, evaluation
team evaluation
group norms

CHAPTER 10
Problem-Solving Steps
problem definition
fact finding
idea finding
criteria selection
solution finding
acceptance finding
Conflict Management
kinds of conflict
supportive and defensive
climates
steps in resolving conflict

Building a Good
Dental Health Team

9

It's 8:00 A.M. and you are in a small waiting room. Joyce, the receptionist, says to you, "The doctor will be with you in a moment." The walls are papered in an ivory grasscloth, the lighting is soft, and the chairs are extremely comfortable. The *National Geographic World Cookbook* attracts your attention. Just as you start to flip through its pages, the dental assistant asks you to come with her to the operatory. There, you are asked to sit in a beige contour chair, the assistant places the napkin around you neck, and the dentist comes in and greets you with a vibrant smile . . . .

You might agree that the office described above would make you feel relaxed and comfortable. Such a pleasant atmosphere is designed to relieve tension and anxiety. It appears so obvious to the patient waiting for a dental appointment. The surroundings are nice, the receptionist and dental assistant are cordial and warm, and the dentist is glad to see you. But what makes them so responsive and cohesive as a group of individuals rendering dental care? Why do you, the patient, perceive that the tasks they perform are so easily accomplished? And *how* are they truly accomplished? Now let us consider how this dental team looks behind the scene.

It's 7:30 A.M. and you accompany Joyce through a side door of the dental office. She immediately turns on the lights, makes sure you are comfortable, and then heads down the back stairs to switch on the air compressor and suction. It all seems so automatic, but so essential for the daily tasks to be per-

167

formed. As she heads toward her desk she stops at the stereo and tunes it in to a mellow station, then proceeds into the laboratory and plugs in the autoclave. She double checks the schedule for the day, which she typed before leaving last evening, and verifies that all the patient records have been pulled. It's now 7:45 A.M., and through the back door comes a cheerful "Good Morning." It is Doris, the dental assistant. She immediately goes to the laboratory to check the schedule, making sure that the trays she prepared before leaving last evening are complete and ready to be placed in the operatories. The phone rings and almost simultaneously another cheerful "Good Morning" comes from the back door. It is Nancy, the dental hygienist. "That was your 8:00 o'clock appointment, Nancy. She has just had an accident and will not be able to make it, so I rescheduled her for the same time next week," explains Joyce. "Is she all right?" "Yes," replies Joyce, "She said not to worry about her." "Well, what needs to be done, Joyce? Shall I help you with the recall system now, or does Doris need me to sharpen instruments?" Then: "Hello, ladies! What's on the agenda for today besides a lunch date with me?" as the dentist rounds the corner. "Good morning, Doctor," the staff chimes, and the day continues.

These individuals probably are a productive and satisfied group of professionals. They appear to work well together. But as we all know, relationships of this kind among individuals aren't easy to achieve. What is it that makes a group of people effective with their patients as well as with one another? What is it that makes an efficient and productive dental health team rendering quality dental care?

Definition of a Dental Health Team

For the purpose of answering these questions, it is appropriate to establish a concrete definition of a working team. Numerous researchers have offered their own definitions, which vary to some degree. However, there are several common elements that must be included in such a definition. It must

1. Comprise fewer than twenty individuals
2. Be task-oriented
3. Have regular interaction at a specific location
4. Be distinguished from other groups and other people
5. Work toward a common goal
6. Have specific job responsibilities assigned to specific individuals

Using these six elements, we can define a dental health team as *a small group of individuals with specific role delineations who are delivering preventive dental services on a regular basis.* There are many qualifiers to this definition, so use it as a basic foundation for the discussion to follow on team building.[1]

BASIC INGREDIENTS FOR A SUCCESSFUL TEAM.   What makes a dental team successful? What qualities do team members possess as individuals and as a group that make them productive and effective in delivering preventive dental treatment? There are four essential ingredients that relate not only to a dental health team, but to any group of people working toward a common goal. Individual team members must

1. Communicate regularly
2. Share in decision-making
3. Have some kind of interdependence with one another
4. Recognize themselves as a *team* needing one another to accomplish their goals[2]

The nature of the dental health team described in the examples beginning this chapter and the way people behave as a team cannot simply be explained in terms of the people who make up the team, nor can the function of the team dynamics be explained simply by the fact that there is a good interpersonal relationship among these individuals. The behavior of the team and how the members work together is affected by the very fact that they communicate with one another and consider themselves a unit in which the members are interdependent in the delivery of dental care. Each member may need the other member for acceptance and a feeling of positive well-being. However, in our earlier example, Joyce, Doris, Nancy, and the doctor constitute an effective team basically because their interdependence relates to the common task of delivering the very best dental care to patients that they can provide.

These four people also meet on a daily basis. Their interaction with one another is at a specific location and a specific time. The four common ingredients cited above must be present within the context of dental health care in order for there to be a productive and effective team.

FACTORS INFLUENCING
DENTAL HEALTH TEAM
EFFECTIVENESS

Most dental health teams are concerned primarily with office productivity, professional satisfaction among the staff members, and the quality of care delivered to patients. Figure 9–1 visually summarizes the relationships among several factors that are influential to the effectiveness and success of many private-practice dental health teams. Three of the five variables which

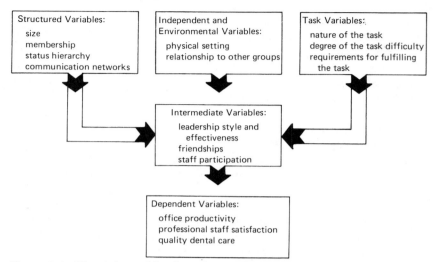

Figure 9-1. Chart of variables that relate to the effectiveness of a dental health team.

specifically relate to the effectiveness of any group of individuals—including a dental team—working toward a common set of goals include

1. Structured variables
2. Independent or environmental variables
3. Task-related variables[3]

The *structured variables* include such things as the size of the dental health team, the staff membership, status hierarchy among group members, and the communication networks within the group. The *independent or environmental variables* refer to the physical setting of the dental office, the environmental factors with which the team lives on a daily basis, and the team's relationship to other working groups of individuals—i.e., the way they differ from other groups of people trying to accomplish a particular task (for example, a group of individuals meeting socially to help a fund-raising activity for a charity as compared with a basketball team playing a game). *Task-related* variables take into account the nature of the work to be done by the team members (i.e., cavity preparation, occlusal adjustment, or soft tissue curettage), the degree of difficulty of the work, and the requirements needed for accomplishing the work (i.e., education and special technical skills, experience, time). These three variables all assist in maximizing the *dependent variables* illustrated in Figure 9-1—office productivity, professional job satisfaction of the staff members, and the quality of dental care rendered to patients.

The *intermediate variables* are influential in terms of the first three, as can be seen in the illustration. Included in the intermediate variables are the leaders of the group and the different leadership styles that emerge among group members, interpersonal relationships within the team, and the role delineation and the participation of the staff in the attainment of the dependent variables. If a dentist understands the importance and mechanics of the structured, environmental, and task-related variables as they relate to his or her office situation, the accomplishment of the dependent variables is not difficult to achieve, because the dentist to a great extent controls the dependent variables in the office environment. Reflect for a moment on the example at the beginning of this chapter. The dentist's first comment to his staff personnel was "Hello, ladies! What's on the agenda for today besides a lunch date with me?" His positive attitude cannot be overlooked and neither can his unexpected invitation for lunch. In this particular situation the dentist is establishing a supportive communication network. An intermediate variable affecting most dental health teams is the leadership style of the designated leader—the dentist. This person is the chief of the team in small private dental offices. He or she hires and fires staff personnel and delineates specific job responsibilities to staff members. (This is not always true, however; in a large urban dental clinic, the business manager may have responsibility for personnel. A receptionist may also have this responsibility in some dental practices.) Leadership styles are important to dental health teams, and will be discussed in more detail later on in this chapter.

Interpersonal relationships among the team members and the distribution of their work responsibilities are intermediate variables affecting the three variables illustrated in Figure 9-1. The dentist can definitely influence the interpersonal relationships among staff members as in the example in the beginning of the chapter. By merely inviting his team to lunch, he creates a social communication network between the people involved and puts communication messages on a social level. Relationships of some kind develop when two or more individuals work together on a daily basis. A dentist's leadership can influence positive and productive relationships. But no one person can control them, as experience has taught us all. Therefore, problems can arise within any dental health team. The way these problems are dealt with may be a result of the dentist's style of leadership, but how *you* deal with them as a member of the team is essential to their resolution. This will be discussed in further detail in Chapter 10.

Staff participation relates not only to the attitude of the individual team members but also to the role delineation placed upon them in the dental office. During conversations which the authors had with dental auxiliaries in private practice, a common feeling kept surfacing: Many of these practicing professionals really did not know what their dentist expected of them, primarily because nothing had been formally written down or said to them by the dentist. They had learned what was expected of them by experiencing positive as well as negative nonverbal and verbal feedback from other team members.

Communication scientists studying group dynamics have found correlations among individual motivation, the office environment, leadership styles, group productivity, and professional staff satisfaction. It is important for you to be conscious of and knowledgable about these factors as a member of a dental health team. They will be discussed later in this chapter as they relate to the establishment of good communication networks in effective working dental teams.[4]

THE NEEDS OF PEOPLE
ON A DENTAL HEALTH TEAM

When asked the question, "What makes yours an effective dental health team?" dental auxiliaries and dentists in a variety of private practice situations, answered as follows:

> The need of belonging. By that I mean the feeling that I am welcome on the team and that the team honestly needs me as a person and not only for my title, experience, and education.
>
> Being understanding and empathetic toward one another and our patients.
>
> The sense of professional worth and value. A feeling that I am essential to the delivery of quality dental care; that without me such a high standard would be more difficult to attain.
>
> Knowing what is expected by the dentist. When I know what I am specifically responsible for doing, then I can work confidently.
>
> Our team is successful, I believe, because we all share in the office planning. We all help in establishing the office policies by which we live and work together on a daily basis.
>
> I think what helps our team work well together is that we feel that we do deliver quality dental care, and are treating our patients with competence.
>
> One factor that helps is the feeling of being challenged. I need to be continually open to new techniques and treatment procedures . . . not knowing everything helps keep me stimulated in my daily work.
>
> Communication!
>
> Respect for ourselves and patients.
>
> Feeling good about ourselves as people helps increase our levels of respect for one another, as well as our ability to communicate.

Being prepared for office procedures. If I did not prepare for the next day the evening before, I would not keep on schedule . . . and that creates tension and anxiety for the dentist, the dental assistant, and the dental hygienist.

Being flexible is the name of the game. If everyone in this office could not bend with the punches, so to speak, we would constantly be on each others' nerves.

Dealing with conflict immediately I truly think helps our team function well together.

We definitely need one another. Each person in this office is essential. We almost fall apart when someone is ill. . . .

Trust and honesty.

To understand these comments, it seems appropriate to again turn to Abraham Maslow's explanation of human motivation as discussed in Chapter 8. According to his theory, an individual's motivation is based on first satisfying the primary physical needs of food, shelter, and clothing. Once these needs are satisfied, the individual's need for security, then social acceptance, then esteem, and finally self-actualization become motivating factors. What needs are being expressed by the dental professionals' comments? Are they expressing more than physiological needs? The answer is obviously yes. They are expressing needs related to self-esteem, the sense of belonging, the ability to communicate, trustworthiness and honesty. One of the things that is important in applying the basic premises of Maslow's theory is to observe and evaluate your own level of needs when you become a member of a dental health team. Be conscious and aware of the motivational factors that affect your role and job responsibilities on a team.

EVOLUTION OF A TEAM

PERCEPTIONS OF SELF AND OTHERS.   Chapter 3 defined perception as a set of assumptions that have developed in an individual through past experiences. In other words, we select, organize, and assign meaning to the many stimuli that affect our daily lives. It is a complex process with many extraneous factors influencing the perceiver's accuracy about another person or experience. The importance of this discussion is to emphasize that perceptions and misperceptions form the foundation of relationships with peers on a dental health team. Being consious of your perceptions and how they develop is vital to your being a positive and effective factor in a team situation. Your perception of yourself as a team member stems from many sources (Figure 3–2 illustrates some of these). However, during conversations with dental auxiliaries in private practice we discovered three additional factors: (1) competency, (2) the respect shown by peers, and (3) influence in the team. The perceptions derived from these influencing factors and many others creates in all of us a frame of reference.

FRAME OF REFERENCE. A person's frame of reference helps to explain his or her behavior in a team and the interpersonal relationships with peers. It is human nature to want to have a feeling of adequacy in our personal frame of reference. Thus, we usually try to behave in a way that will enhance us in the eyes of others. For example, in the example at the beginning of this chapter, when her 8 o'clock patient canceled, the dental hygienist offered to assist the receptionist on the recalls or help the dental assistant by sharpening instruments. One might conclude that she is comfortable with her frame of reference and self-perception, and therefore feels good about herself; this in turn enables her to be flexible and comfortable assisting team members with their job responsibilities.

Teams working together toward common goals in some way create their own frame of reference. This may occur subconsciously; but it stems from the variables illustrated in Figure 9–1. Many influencing elements play a role in developing their perception of their dental health team. They may perceive themselves as productive and efficient, or think that they are overworked and underpaid. So what happens is that the team gradually compiles a working profile or perception of themselves. As the self-fulfilling prophecy discussed in Chapter 3 postulates, the team actually will perform in terms of the way they see themselves and their responsibilities in the dental office. The familiar saying "You are what you think you are" becomes a reality once again.

INFLUENCE OF ROLES. Roles also emerge on teams basically through individual team members' self-perceptions as well as others' perceptions of them. Roles influence self-perceptions, and relate appropriately to the behavior pattern of the entire team. The establishment of identities and roles are necessary in all working teams, but understanding their influence on the communication networks within the team and with individuals is also very important.

EFFECTIVE BEHAVIORS. Small-group dynamics have been studied for years. The success of a group, and for our purposes we are referring to a dental health team in a private-practice situation, depends on many factors. In discussions with practicing professionals on working dental teams, we have come to believe that there are behaviors that the members of these teams possess that make them effective and productive in their work. We do not intend to say that these are the *only* qualities necessary for small-group effectiveness; we are only suggesting that these behaviors seem to be consistently present in dental health teams that communicate and work well together. As you approach the challenge of being a member of a dental health team, you can develop the behavioral skills listed below that you already practice, or begin to devise a plan to improve the behaviors that you need development.

COGNITIVE BEHAVIOR SKILLS

Initiative Do not merely react to others. Do not wait to be asked. Reach out to others and offer your assistance. Nancy, the dental hygienist in the example at the beginning of this chapter, displayed initiative.

Flexibility Be willing, during daily office routines, to compromise with others' actions, procedures, and suggestions.

Congruency Strive to have your verbal and nonverbal behavior send consistent messages. One receptionist said that an excellent criterion for determining the level of trust and honesty on her team was the fact that members of the team would say inside the group the things they would say outside the group privately to friends, spouses, etc. However, appropriate timing is an element that should not be underestimated.

Ability to Speak for Self Deal with problems and conflicts immediately. Do not hold grudges or misunderstandings inside. Speak for yourself, so as not to polarize the team. Use "I" rather than "you," "she," or "we." Be concrete and specific in your interactions.

Responsibility Be on time for work. Be reliable. If you say you will do it, then by all means do it, even if you have to stay an hour later. Keep on schedule by being prepared.

Self-Respect and Genuineness Be yourself. Do not pretend to be someone you are not. Be honest with yourself, about yourself, your abilities, strengths, etc. Be sincere. Practice your personal and professional code of ethics. Respect that standard and maintain excellence. These qualities will help to establish a climate of trust and open communication on a dental health team.

Openness Be open to new ideas and ways of doing things in the office. Do not think that you know it all. Listen to what others have to say to you and learn from them.

Empathy Put your feet into the other person's shoes. Be conscious of his or her problems and emotions. Be

Pride

understanding. Be patient. Treat others as you would want to be treated yourself. Learn to listen. Feel glad to be part of the team. Take pride in how the team communicates and delivers dental care.

COMMUNICATION NETWORKS

Throughout this chapter the term "communication network" has been frequently mentioned. It was first illustrated in Figure 9–1 as a structured variable influencing the effectiveness of a dental health team. Communication networks need considerable attention here because of their great influence on the effectiveness and productivity of the entire team. For clarity, we shall refer to a communication network in a dental health team as *a number of individuals who persistently interact with one another on a daily basis in certain communication patterns*. When we discuss communication networks, we also imply that the individuals who communicate a great deal with one another establish their network out of a mutual concern. In the instance of a dental health team, that mutual concern would be the delivery of quality dental care, as well as office producitivity and professional job satisfaction. Communication networks within a dental health team are not always predictable, because they continually change.[5]

System Effects

Communication networks also provide an understanding of individual members' behavior on the team. Communication scientists refer to this as *system effects*. System effects are the influences of others on a team on the behavior of an individual member of the team.[6] For example, Nancy, the dental hygienist, offered to assist Joyce, the receptionist, on the recalls during her cancellation time. Most likely, if Nancy gets behind schedule some day, Joyce will be willing to help clean the instruments and disinfect the operatory while Nancy prepares her instruments for her next patient. If Nancy, for example, only wants to be responsible for her own patients and instruments, the rest of the team will likely respond to her in a similar manner. As the common saying goes, "You get back as much as you give."

Types of Networks

Through research, communication scientists have also concluded that there are three distinguishing concepts relating to the communication networks in small working groups. As they relate to a dental health team, these concepts are:

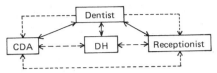

Figure 9–2. Total system communication network.

1. *Total system communication networks*, which are the communication patterns that develop among all the team members in a dental office.
2. *Personal communication networks*, the patterns that individual members establish with other individuals on the team.[7]
3. *Cliques*, the subsystems that consist of members who interact more frequently with one another than with other team members.

TOTAL SYSTEM NETWORKS.   The total system communication network is illustrated in Figure 9–2. It is important to note that this particular example is a formal system communication network. In a dental health team the dentist, within the formal communication network, is the designated leader. Informal communication networks are always involved in any group of individuals, however. This is also true on a dental health team. Informal communication networks are usually subordinate to the formal structure, but not always. For example, one dental hygienist in private practice stated that the dentist on her team had no idea how much money he made a year. The receptionist was responsible for all his professional and personal finances. She ordered the office supplies, wrote out the pay checks for the entire team, decided on office policies. The dentist in this particular situation was by organization and structure the designated leader, but he had delegated his power to the receptionist. Other informal communication networks within a dental health team relate quite specifically to the roles the team members play. Later in this chapter, the types of roles that occur in small groups, and their influences on the team's total system communication network, will be discussed.

PERSONAL NETWORKS.   Each of us has a network of friends with whom we consistently interact. This personal communication network creates a comfortable environment for most of us. An individual's personal communication network can reflect on his or her behavior patterns in a team situation. Figure 9–3 illustrates the personal communication of Individual A. To fully understand Individual A's behavior in a team situation we would have to analyze more in depth the other individuals' characteristics in his network (Individuals I, II, and III). For our purposes in this discussion, such an analysis is not relevant. Figure 9–4 also demonstrates how Individual A's personal communication network comprising of friends I, II, and III grows into a larger network, which includes their friends and their friends' friends.

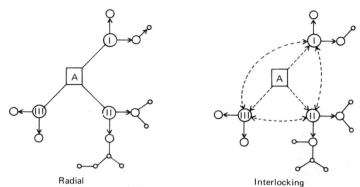

Radial   Interlocking

Figure 9–3. Personal communication network.

Personal communication networks have been more specifically defined by Rogers and Agarwala-Rogers, two communication scientists who have divided the personal communication network into a personal radial network and a personal interlocking network. A radial network is one in which Individual A interacts directly with his friends I, II, and III, and Individual A's friends do not interact with one another. This is demonstrated in Figure 9–3. An interlocking personal network is one in which Individual A's friends I, II, and III interact with one another. This is also illustrated in Figure 9–3.[8]

CLIQUES.   Cliques are identified among the members of a dental health team on the basis of which individuals communicate most with one another. These cliques are then superimposed in the formal organization of the dental team. A simulated clique is illustrated in Figure 9–4. Consider the illustration as a large urban dental clinic. Four dentists have four different private practices within one building. Each manages his own practice, dental assistant, and

Figure 9–4. Diagrammatic model of cliques.

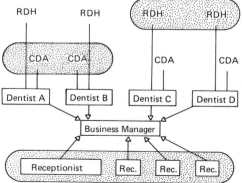

dental hygienist. They hire a business manager to be responsible for the fiscal aspects of all their practices, the records, ordering of supplies, and receptionists. Within this formal organization emerge the following cliques: (1) the receptionists, who work side by side on a daily basis and eat lunch together on a regular basis; (2) the dental assistants from dentist A and B, who went to school together and have only been working five months; (3) the dental hygienists in doctor C and D's offices, who are taking a special course on soft tissue curettage at night from a local periodontist. Cliques form for a variety of reasons in any group of individuals. They can be positive influences on a group, as well as negative. The importance of a clique in our context is that it relates specifically to the communication networks of the entire dental health team.

Communication networks are the threads that hold a dental health team together. They are complex and extremely versatile in any given dental practice. As you prepare to become a member of a dental health team, your awareness of communication networks will assist you in your communication and interpersonal relationships with members of the team. By no means has this brief discussion covered the discipline of small-group communication networks in detail. We have tried to make you aware of the existence of networks and to show how they relate to the organization of a dental health team.

BUILDING A SUCCESSFUL DENTAL HEALTH TEAM

As we have mentioned previously in this chapter, a dental health team's effectiveness is influenced by three dependent variables: *office productivity, professional job satisfaction,* and *quality dental services.* But what makes one group of dental professionals productive and another not as productive? What makes one football team a winner over another team? Skill and talent have much to do with the success of any team. But always important to the team are the communication networks *within* the team. These networks make effectiveness and success possible because it builds cohesiveness. *Cohesiveness* refers to the ability of the team to work together as one unit toward a common set of goals. It exists when each member of the team works for the entire team and not for personal gain. Think again of the example beginning this chapter. Do you think the individuals on that particular team worked cohesively? Their cohesiveness was demonstrated in several ways. Joyce, for example, came early to prepare the office for the day. Doris made sure the operatory trays for the dental procedures were correct and ready to go for the dentist. Nancy voluntarily offered her assistance to both Doris and Joyce.

Members of cohesive groups generally take initiative and help one another. They see that the workload is distributed evenly. Cohesiveness is related closely to a group's morale. Do the members like one another? Do they spend time and effort in behalf of the entire group? The more cohesive, the more open are the communication networks within the group. In turn, more feedback is given and received. In a cohesive dental health team each member knows what is expected, and feels respected and secure in his or her professional responsibilities. Members of a cohesive group understand that disagreements will arise from time to time due to the constant pressures of a busy dental practice—but they know it is O.K. for their "togetherness" to fluctuate from day to day. However, they also know that they have something common at stake, and that it takes each one of them to deliver the dental care to their patients.

Guidelines for Achieving Cohesiveness

You may be wondering how that team in the initial example beginning this chapter reached such a high level of cohesiveness. It is obvious that groups of individuals, each of whom comes from many areas and backgrounds do not inherently have cohesiveness when they meet. Below are listed ways in which dental health teams can achieve cohesiveness:

1. Identify your group. Talk about your team in terms of "we" and "us." Discuss how "our" team can be better organized, how "we" can manage our time better, how "we" can keep on schedule.
2. Create some kind of tradition. Highly cohesive families gather together for celebration on holidays and for other special occasions. The same is true for cohesive dental teams. Some have annual parties. Other teams plan to attend at least two dental continuing education programs a year. Tradition helps add meaning and loyalty to the team as a whole.
3. Don't worry about who gets the credit for getting the job done as long as the entire group benefits and succeeds. Think *teamwork*. Stress the importance of each member's responsibility on the team. Delivering high-quality dental care cannot be done by the dentist alone, or the dental hygienist alone. Every individual is needed to render dental services to patients in the most effective, efficient way possible.
4. Learn to recognize the potential and positive effects of other team members. Verbally compliment them. Recognize them in some fashion. Encourage professional involvement in school screening or Dental Health Week. Being praised for the importance of the contribution to the team creates a great deal of personal motivation and pride.
5. Know what you as a team want to accomplish. Set some clear, definable goals. They can be long-range, as well as short-range. Reaching goals is exciting and can enhance the team's morale.

6. Provide "rewards." Reaching team goals is definitely a reward and a feather in the cap. A dentist can create tradition, stress teamwork, compliment his staff, encourage goals by recognizing with some kind of reward. The dentist at the beginning of this chapter invited his team to lunch, providing a positive, spontaneous reward. A reward such as that definitely adds to a team's morale and cohesiveness. Auxiliaries who have leadership roles can do the same thing. A reward from the dentist or any team member is really just a "thank you" for a job well done or a gesture of appreciation.

7. Live by the golden rule—treat others as you want to be treated. Individuals on the dental health team are people. As we all know so well, people are not perfect and have many faults. Thus, learning to compromise and forgive and forget truly adds to the cohesiveness of a team.

COMMUNICATION EXERCISE 9-1

Below is an excerpt from a conversation with a Certified Dental Assistant. List the cohesive actions demonstrated by the RDH and the CDA. Do you think they had a good working relationship?

> . . . The dental hygienist in our office usually took her own bitewings, but sometimes when she would get behind schedule, I would take them for her. Then if I were really busy, she would help me out by taking X-rays or assisting the dentist. We were working with each other, not against each other. If she didn't have a patient she would ask me how to set up the trays and clean instruments. She didn't just sit around. It was great when I came out of the operatory after assisting the dentist—the jobs were all done. If she were busy and we had a cancellation, I would assist her during polishing or suction when she used the cavitron.

Are there any additional cohesive actions? List them below.

1.
2.
3.
4.

Consider the following excerpt from a conversation with a CDA. What actions could this CDA take to make the dental office environment more cohesive? List them below.

> I was in an office where the receptionist kept saying "Oh, I'll do that." She sort of tried to take over the dental assisting responsibilities

(continued)

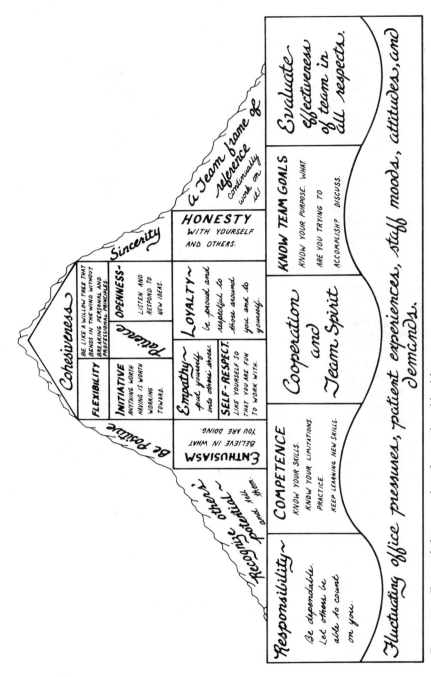

Figure 9–5. Essential elements of a cohesive dental health team.

182

COMMUNICATION EXERCISE 9-1 *(Contd)*

sometimes. I felt subordinate to her in many respects. I always kept thinking that she would shine and the rest of the staff wouldn't look as good in the dentist's eyes. I didn't say anything to the dentist. I just tried to do the best job I could do at dental assisting.

1.
2.
3.
4.

Creating a cohesive dental health team is a definite challenge. Relationships with people always involve struggles. But overcoming the obstacles and struggles together as a team will benefit each member's well-being and make each one a better person.[9]

THE DYNAMICS OF THE DENTAL HEALTH TEAM

As a member of a dental health team, it is important to be conscious of what you do, and the choices you must make, because in many instances your actions will have an impact upon the other members of the team. The potential of a team stems from a variety of sources: the diverse backgrounds of the members; the specialized skills, education, and experiences in other dental offices. If these are combined effectively, a cohesive team can develop. But these differences in the team members can also create differences in their perceptions concerning what the team is trying to accomplish and their own role on the team. Thus, it is essential for team members to ask themselves the following questions:

1. What are we trying to accomplish?
2. How can we best achieve our goals?
3. Where do we want to go as a team?

RESOLVING DIFFERENCES. Delivering comprehensive dental care is obviously not a simple task. Consequently, the individuals on the team do not have the same assumptions concerning the team goals and their role responsibilities. Without a shared understanding of these things, conflicts can arise. Consider the following example:

> I've had several dental hygienists who only wanted to do hygiene. We talked about the fact that they were a vital component in the entire machinery of this office. In fact, how they did their jobs literally affected the way I could do mine. But all they wanted to do was dental hygiene. They did not want to help call patients or update the recall system. We weren't on the same wave length. My idea and their idea of their function in this office were two totally different things.

The danger illustrated here is that the dental hygienist and the dentist are in conflict. How to deal with conflict and resolve differences will be discussed in the following chapter. But the point to remember is that there will always be some lack of agreement among members of a dental health team. The degree of congruence or incongruence is what will make the difference between a team being successful, having initiative to get things done, creating cohesiveness, and having a feeling of togetherness. Establishing goals together as a group is a positive step toward building an effective team, and equally important is the clear delineation of professional roles. To achieve these goals, ask yourself the following two questions:

1. What are my reasons for being a member of this team?
2. What is the entire team trying to accomplish?

ESTABLISHING TEAM GOALS.   The accomplishment of goals for an effective dental health team requires a leader who makes sure that things get done in the dental office. The fact that you are a member of a *team* means that no one individual on that team has the knowledge and skills necessary to render total dental care to patients. In order to deliver preventive services, therefore, the team needs organization, coordination, and allocation of responsibilities. It is important for a dental health team to have a leader who will keep the group interacting and functioning together to create office productivity, job satisfaction, and quality dental care. No one person can accomplish the team goals, and neither can one person be responsible for leading the team in all situations.

Leadership Styles

Leadership can be formal or informal in style and function. For the purposes of this discussion, *leadership* consists of positive communication by an individual which motivates the dental health team to actively work toward its common goals.[10] A leader in a team situation is someone who helps structure the group, has knowledge and expertise in delivering comprehensive dental health care, and is a model on whom other team members can emulate and pattern their professionalism.

COMMUNICATION EXERCISE 9–2

Indicate whether you agree or disagree with the following qualities that are listed below for a leader on a dental health team.

	AGREE	DISAGREE
1. Seeks ideas	———	———
2. Knowledgeable about dentistry and business	———	———
3. Influential	———	———
4. Mature	———	———
5. Assertive	———	———
6. Conflict resolver	———	———
7. Motivator	———	———
8. Open communicator	———	———
9. Creates a positive climate in the office	———	———
10. Evaluator	———	———
11. Fair	———	———
12. Empathetic	———	———
13. Good listener	———	———
14. Rational	———	———
15. Nonjudgmental	———	———

In conversations with dental auxiliaries in private practice, the authors found that a primary element in their feeling of team cohesiveness was the fact that they had leadership. The leadership in many circumstances was not formal, but informal in nature. That is, the dentist in the formal structure of the team was the designated leader, but in reality was not the person who actually provided the leadership for the group in many situations. Qualities of leadership that the auxiliaries expressed indicated that team leaders, either formal or informal, (1) possessed knowledge of dentistry and business; (2) were self-motivated; (3) were fair in their dealings with other people on the team; (4) displayed maturity; (4) openly communicated and verbalized their thoughts; (5) were assertive and influential with other members on the team; (6) showed authority by resolving conflicts; and (7) created a positive work climate and environment.

Leadership is a complex process of human interaction on a dental health team. It is influenced by the goals of the team, the nature of the group, the members' needs, the nature of the formal designated leader, the various situations in which the team operates, the needs and characteristics of the team members themselves, and much more. A leader on a dental health team emerges through the group process as a result of personal qualities and traits, as well as the person's contribution to the fulfillment of the team's needs and goals. As the leader of a dental health team emerges, so does a particular *style of leadership.* In personal interviews with dental health team members, the following four leadership styles were commonly found existing in their particular team and private-practice situations:

1. *Authoritative.* This particular style is characterized by the designated leader, the dentist, being in total control of the office. That person "rules the roost," so to speak.
2. *Consultive.* A consultive leader seeks the opinions and suggestions of other team members, and then makes decisions and office policies. Usually the dentist was noted as the primary leader in this style.
3. *Democratic.* This style of leadership is characterized by the group process. This leadership is present in dental offices that have regular staff meetings to decide procedure, activities, policies, etc.
4. *Laissez-faire.* This style indicates complete freedom among the team members. No one particular person, formally or informally, emerges as a leader in this particular dental office situation.[11]

AUTHORITATIVE.   An authoritative leader is a person who is the decision-maker and problem-solver. This style is characterized by the designated leader (e.g., the dentist) being in total control. That person "rules the roost," and others on the team are subordinate. In this leadership style, everyone needs to be very clear about his or her roles and assigned tasks. As long as each does the assigned tasks, communication follows direct lines understood by all. When someone tries to make a shift in role or task boundary, it could cause friction on the team.

CONSULTATIVE.   This leadership style is evident when one person makes the decisions, but with a "the buck stops here" philosophy. However, this type of leader listens actively to others and recognizes the value of other ideas than his or her own. A dental hygienist might be taken very seriously by a consultative-leader-type dentist when the RDH makes a suggestion about patient relations, for example. The leader using this style credits everyone with having worthwhile contributions.

DEMOCRATIC.   In democratic leadership, many viewpoints are welcome and decisions are made after discussion, dialogue, and perhaps even debate. Decisions are made either by consensus or by a vote. The leader may be less vocal than in other styles, but he or she maintains control over the *process* and makes sure that the method of decision making is followed. In this process, the leader tends to have a low profile and does not need to "take charge" in daily procedures.

LAISSEZ-FAIRE.   There is complete freedom and no designated or "official" leader in laissez-faire-type leadership. Everyone does what seems to be needed at the time. People who have worked together for a long time may be able to operate this way; other groups may become frustrated by a lack of formal structure and unclear guidelines. Leaders may emerge from any part of the team and eventually enforce one of the other three leadership styles.

GROUP ORGANIZATION.   Lee Thayer suggests that what is organized in a business group is not people, but the *relationship* of information-flow systems and conversation centers.[12] Thus, it would be the task of a leader of a dental team to organize a system which allows the information received from each person to be acknowledged and developed in the fulfillment of daily tasks. The leader chooses information, which comes from many members of the team, and decides what to do with it. The style of leadership, as discussed above, determines how the team is run. In a dental office, if the leader were a dentist operating by a domestic-consensus pattern, he or she would make very clear to the other team members (receptionist, dental assistants, dental hygienists, bookkeepers, etc.) how they are to give and receive (process and respond to) information throughout the day. The dentist, in this case, would also be the person who calls staff meetings and sees to it that ideas, grievances, problems, and other information is processed so that appropriate action occurs.

As situations change in the dental office, so do the leaders and their leadership styles. Many dentists are team leaders simply by virtue of their position and education. On the other hand, the informal leader emerges within the team basically because of personal traits and qualities. Depending on a multitude of variables, each leader is vital to the entire team's communication network and cohesiveness—because without leadership, groups lose direction and responsibility for their goals.

Roles

As we have mentioned previously, specific *roles* emerge among members of any dental health team. They emerge within the formal communication network as well as the informal communication system network of the team. For example, in one group of people you may be a take-charge person who gets things moving and creates action among the group members. In another situation and in another group of people, you may be well liked and dependable, but not a leader. In a third situation, with totally different people, you may be a companion, a good listener, and a compromiser. A person changes roles from group to group, and your characteristics within each group are to some extent determined by the people around you.

In order to determine the roles that are played by individual team members, researchers of small-group communication have looked at the self-perception of people within the small group. Think back for a moment on the discussion of self-perception and personal frame of reference in this chapter. To a great extent, your feelings about yourself in a given situation determine how you will approach the particular situation. Your personal self-perceptions and expectations correlate directly with your personal frame of reference, from which you operate and interact with others. These, in turn, are the threads to the responsive roles you play on a dental health team.

Role Ambiguity.   Lois has worked for Dr. X for eighteen years as receptionist and dental assistant. During the past year, Dr. X has taken an associate in the office because he is reaching retirement age. Lois has always made Dr. X's office run smoothly and with little frustration. Keeping on schedule with patients and being prepared are some of the keys to her success. When the new dentist arrived in the office, he hired a young woman to be his dental assistant. She has had no formal dental assistant training. Being confident of her work responsibilities and of herself, Lois knows she can guide the new employee. But how much? Lois knows how to make the office run efficiently, but, in her words, "I do not want to throw too much at the new assistant at one time for several reasons. First of all, I think I might come across too pushy and know-it-all. Second, I do not want to alienate myself on an interpersonal level with her." Lois knows what her role has been in relation to Dr. X. Obviously, her personal self-perception in her role has been adequate, or she and the doctor would not have been a successful team for so many years. But now she is not feeling comfortable in her approach with the new assistant. She is not confident of the role she should be playing. Does she tell the young woman everything she needs to know about the office, or does she just offer suggestions when asked? No one has given her any direction, and she feels ambiguous and uncertain in her role related to the new assistant.

Well-defined roles, as we can see from the above example, help members of a dental health team to create positive perceptions about themselves and their frame of reference. Knowing what is expected of you influences your behavior as well as enabling you to anticipate the behavior of another person. Lois knows, before the new dentist even asks for an instrument in a dental procedure what instrument he will want. But now she finds herself in a new role—one that is *not* specifically defined—in terms of the new assistant. She now feels role ambiguity. This feeling saps an individual's energy and can lead to lower office productivity, job dissatisfaction, and lower quality of dental care. The symptoms of role ambiguity appear when a person starts asking the following questions:

1. What should I do?
2. Do other team members think I am doing what is expected of me?

3. What should other team members be doing?
4. Are there things I cannot get done because someone else does not seem to be doing the job?

Several approaches are useful in dealing with role ambiguity. When you become a member of a dental health team, ask your employer for an office procedures manual. (We acknowledge that although office procedures manuals are usually thought about and discussed, the majority of private dental practices do not have them.) Discuss the goals of the office with the dentist and other team members. Ask for a job description in writing, so that you know exactly what is expected of you. Also, ask about the job responsibilities of other team members. Be confident about what is expected of you by all members on the team. This will help insure your job satisfaction and productivity and avoid conflicts with other team members concerning role delineation.

For example, Marsha, a registered dental hygienist, works for a dentist only on Mondays. She relates the following story of role ambiguity and conflict. On one occasion the dentist asked her, "Marsha, why doesn't Pat clean up the laboratory?" Later, Pat told Marsha, "The doctor is expecting far too much from me. I don't see why Jan, the receptionist, can't do some more around here." Still later, Jan asked, "Marsha—can I talk with you a moment before you leave? I want to know why Pat has been so on edge lately. She has been so aloof and distant. I think she thinks I am not doing my job." What is Marsha's role in this office? No one seems to know hers, or theirs either.

Not only are the role delineations in this particular office unclear, but conflicting perceptions of roles can be noted by the dentist, Jan, and Pat. Looking at the example more specifically in terms of role conflict, three facts are apparent. There is (1) role conflict—this is evident with Pat in her relationship with the dentist and the receptionist. There is also (2) role conflict between members' perceptions of others' responsibilities. And there is (3) the role conflict that arises from Pat's being overworked. In the following chapter we will deal with role conflicts more specifically. It is important to know now that the inevitable outcome of role ambiguity in a dental office between members of the team is personal conflict. Role ambiguity and conflict do not add to dental health team cohesiveness. Without a feeling of togetherness, the team's goals cannot be effectively accomplished.

Role Evaluation

One way to understand how a group works is to evaluate the roles the members play. This will help each member see why the group works as it does. Understanding, as in all aspects of communication, is the first prerequisite for making changes or for strengthening the current situation. What roles are there in working groups? Basically there are three kinds: (1) task roles, (2) maintenance roles, and (3) individual roles. Knowing what these three kinds of roles are will help you analyze your own role on the dental team, and know where to make changes, if necessary, in your own behavior. How you behave affects how others behave.

TASK ROLES.   These are the roles that function to "get the job done." The goal of a dental team is to provide quality preventive dental care for a certain public group—the patients. Each activity performed to meet this goal in each individual case is a task, and many people may be involved. Look for the following task roles in the daily work of your team or in staff meetings:

Initiator	This person is the one who gets a topic out in front of others for discussion. "Well, doctor, I don't know if you've noticed how often the receptionist has been overscheduling Lucille, but it's causing some problems which I think we ought to deal with." This person has initiated discussion on a specific problem. He or she may not have the solution, but does recognize a need and gets the problem into the open so that it can be solved.
Information-Seeker	This person asks for factual data and objective information which relates directly to the task. In response to the initiator's statement above, the information-seeker might say, "That could be a problem; how many patients does the receptionist try to give to Lucille during a day, as a general rule?" No judgment is intended, simply an acknowledgement of what the initiator has observed and an attempt to learn more specifics about it.
Information-Giver	This person provides factual information related to the task: "Lucille seems to be getting anywhere from six to seven patients between 8 o'clock and noon, then it slacks off after lunch." Feelings and judgmental opinions are not a part of this role.
Clarifier	The clarifier interprets the information, and explains what it means, perhaps in a technical way or in an informed way that will help the group accomplish a task. "This many appointments in the morning means that patients arriving on time at 9 o'clock often have to wait an hour to see the hygienist, which in turn affects how they relate to the hygienist. Patients get mad at Lucille,

and this begins to hinder Ludy's relationship with them as the morning grows longer. Also, by noon, Lucy still has patients to see and sometimes has to skip lunch in order to get back on schedule at 1 o'clock."

Summarizer This type of person lists all the important facts and opinions that have been given so far, helping everyone keep the whole picture in mind and not get bogged down on one item. "So far, these are the things I've heard stated . . . ."

Synthesizer The person who takes the summary and all the various comments and puts all the information into a general statement of where the group is at that moment. This keeps the group on track. This person does not take sides, nor does he or she try to create a debate situation by pointing out extreme differences. Ideally, the task will be resolved by consensus, not by debate, and the synthesizer tries to bring the various parts together into a whole statement with which most members can agree. "Now what I think we are saying is that the receptionist is giving Lucille more patients in the morning than she can handle with adequate attention, and this is creating tension between the patients and Lucy as well as sometimes keeping her from lunch. Is this accurate?"

Idea-Giver The idea-giver offers ideas about how the problem should be solved. Ideas are not dogmatic statements or "the only right solution," but rather possibilities. This person helps move the group toward the task. "One way to solve this might be for Lucy and the receptionist to talk about what a fair appointment schedule would look like on paper."

Evaluator Such a person gives the pros and cons of possible solutions. If this occurs after summaries, ideas, and consensus statements have been given, it likely will help achieve the task. If evaluation occurs too soon, the group could polarize or move into a time-consuming debate. "It seems to me that if we think about taking fewer patients in the morning, the result might be beneficial. On the other hand, . . ."

There are other task roles, but these are the most common found on dental health teams.

MAINTENANCE ROLES.   These roles function to keep the group going, no matter what the task (and sometimes even if there is no task). These deal with relationships—between group members as they decide *how* they will carry on their business. The following maintenance roles are typical:

Harmonizer	This person tries to keep relationships working in a cooperative rather than a defensive manner. A person taking this role is particularly helpful if individuals in the team tend to pair off, or argue and bicker instead of moving on toward a task. An example might be, "I can see that there are two of you with strong opinions about the matter. It would help us if we can find some points you both have in common that relate to the goal we are all working toward." Hoever, a harmonizer may possibly hinder constructive conflict which may need to be dealt with honestly.
Gatekeeper	The person undertaking this role controls information flow.[13] In a staff meeting, such a person might say, "I think we've heard enough ideas. Let's see if we can't find one or two to work on and resolve this problem." In a dental office in which there are few or no regular staff meetings, a gatekeeper might be one who tells one party what another has said. A dental assistant might tell the dentist, for example, that the hygienist is uncomfortable about the receptionist's overscheduling.
Rule-Giver	The person in this role reminds the group from time to time what the guidelines are for the discussion at hand. Or she or he might offer rules by which information should flow within the office staff if decisions are to be made in an acceptable manner. For example, one dental assistant might say to another, "Instead of telling me about that, you should tell Dr. _____, because he's really the one who has to make a decision about that," or, in a staff meeting, "We agreed to discuss this for 10 minutes and it's time now to try to find an answer to the problem."

Maintenance roles of harmonizer, gatekeeper, and rule-giver are the primary roles that function to keep the group working. There are others, including that of "climate-sensor"; a person in this role senses the mood or climate of the group and does much the same thing with group feelings as the synthesizer does with information. This person might say, "We seem to be getting tired; I wonder if we could take a break for a few minutes." Knowing this and other maintenance roles will help you do those things which you may sense would help your group function smoothly.

INDIVIDUAL ROLES.　　Whereas task and maintenance roles relate to the group itself, individual roles are those which people have for themselves. Such roles match our self-concept and express our uniqueness in the group. Again, there are many such roles, but here are a few you might recognize, in terms of yourself or others.

Cynic	The cynic finds very little value in any ideas, on a regular basis, and generally has little hope for workable solutions: "Oh, I've heard *that* idea before!"
Clown	The person undertaking this role makes light of everything. Sometimes this helps relieve tensions; sometimes clownish behavior is so irrelevant that it covers up real problems or makes conflict seem superficial: "What do you mean, we're too busy? Don't *all* CDAs hobble around with bags under their eyes and out of breath, like this?"
Marcher to Different Drummer	This person seems to be on an entirely different track than the rest of the group, and may be independent to the point of being actually not part of the team: "What did you say? Oh, there's a patient waiting? Oops—didn't know it was this late—I was thinking about an idea I have about . . . ."
Silent Loner	This type of person speaks very seldom and minds his or her own business. This role does affect the group and nonverbal messages play a strong part in the information-flow process. This person may really want to be asked for an opinion; or, may just want to work and go home: "(Silence.)"
Mother (Father)	The person whose role behavior typifies that of a parent looks out for everyone else and offers proverbial advice for other's welfare, and may even offer to help others with their work. In a staff meeting, when there is a discussion, this person may be looking out for those who need a coffee refill. The "parent" type may be an easy person for others to confide in. A lot of power could reside in relationships with this person if he or she also has task roles that get problems solved. However, it is a role that can easily be overplayed: "Never mind,

	dear. Don't you worry about it. Let me take care of things."
Blocker	This person likes to kill ideas which others offer: "We *can't* do that! It's been *tried* before. It *never* works! That's the silliest idea I've ever heard."

If you can identify your own roles in a group and feel that you are making a positive contribution, then you know that you probably are doing what is best for you. On the other hand, if you recognize that the effect on the group is not constructive when you take on certain tasks, maintenance, or individual roles, you will be better able to make changes in the roles you undertake. Further, if you are a group leader, identifying who on the team plays dominant roles will help you manage the group more efficiently. More will be said about problem solving and conflict resolution in the next chapter. However, if you try to identify the roles we have mentioned in this chapter each time you work with a group of people, you will begin to develop the skill of sensing the direction in which discussions will go and why the whole organization works the way it does. With this skill, you can make personal changes to help communication system networks flow even better.

Questions for Team Evaluation

Periodically, a team needs to take time together as a group and *evaluate* their goals, work productivity, professional job satisfaction, and quality of dental care that they are rendering to patients. They need to discuss things in a staff meeting. The following questions are helpful in such a context:

1. What are our goals as a team this year?
2. What do we want to do in the next six months as a team?
3. Are we getting things done in the office?
4. Could we get them done in a more efficient manner?
5. What are our perceptions of ourselves as a team?
6. Do our patients like us?
7. How could we be a better team?
8. Are job roles defined explicitly?
9. Is everyone comfortable with their place on the team?
10. Are we knowledgeable on the most current dental research and concepts?
11. Are we giving our patients the best possible care?
12. Are we practicing what we preach to our patients?
13. What personal conflicts need to be resolved?
14. What is the cause of any existing conflicts?
15. What positive steps can we take as a team to relieve stress and tension?
16. Do we have a good feeling about ourselves? Are we a cohesive group?

Being honest in an evaluative process is difficult. Members of a team must be conscious of others' feelings and emotions. But criticism is important for growth in many instances and particularly true when a team's efforts directly affect other human beings. Proceed with caution during a team evaluation meeting; be empathetic toward others; do not judge by actions alone; but above all, be honest.

Group Norms

The job responsibilities of the members of a dental health team are very specialized. As job responsibilities develop and become part of the total systems communication network, another process occurs simultaneously. This process concerns the formation of the standard operating procedures by which the team operates. Communication scientists call these norms. *Group norms* are the nonverbal and verbal "rules" which influence the actions of the team members.[14]

All dental health teams evolve specific norms. Some are written formally—for example, "Dental health team members must be in the office by 8:00 A.M., wearing a uniform." Quite often however, the most influential norms are unwritten. For example, a dental assistant related: "We never disagree with the dentist, and we always address him as Doctor." These norms are informal, unwritten, but they have evolved and been agreed to, perhaps subconsciously, by the team members.

A dental health team's sense of identity, loyalty of the team members, and feeling of cohesiveness relate directly to the group norms established in the office. An individual's level of productivity in the team is influenced, to a great extent, by his or her acceptance of the group norms. The norms developed within a dental health team occur in three areas, involving the social, the procedural, and the task dimensions of a team.[15] The *social dimension* in which norms develop refer to the way the team works together—for example, in terms of their chosen vocabulary and manner of dress. The *procedural dimension* of group norms involves the formality of the group—do members, for example, address one another by first names? It also involves the organizational structure of the team and the ladder of authority. The *task dimension* of group norms develops around the goals and purposes of the team.

Dental health teams should realize that the norms set by the group, agreed upon by individual members, are influential factors affecting how the group works together. Norms are of particular importance to new members on a team because the new member usually needs to learn the group's existing standards in order to work with others in a cooperative way. Group norms can change, if and when group members decide there is a need for a change. A new team member may be the first to recognize the need for a change because he or she has not been so deeply involved with or loyal to existing conditions. Being conscious of the norms in your group will help you to be able to evaluate their value and importance. Remember that norms exist in *all* working groups and are extremely influential in terms of team members' behavior and the success of the team.

COMMUNICATION EXERCISE 9-3

The following statements reflect norms that are likely to exist in private dental offices and on dental health teams. Check if you think they represent formal and informal norms established by the teams. Add additional norms that you have observed in action on a dental health team of which you have been a member.

	FORMAL	INFORMAL
1. "All patients are called by their proper names—i.e., Mr. Jones, Ms. Rogers."	_____	_____
2. "The dentist is always addressed as Doctor."	_____	_____
3. "We always call patients to remind them of their appointment."	_____	_____
4. "During cancellations I try to help with recalls or instrument sharpening."	_____	_____
5. "First appointments are scheduled for 8:00 A.M. so we try to be in by 7:45 A.M. at the latest."	_____	_____
6. "I have 45 minutes for lunch, but we all take turns rotating so that the phone is covered at all times."	_____	_____
7. "A personal code of ethics is maintained."	_____	_____
8. "It is O.K. to make mistakes."	_____	_____
9. "We deal with problems immediately."	_____	_____
10. "No one chews gum."	_____	_____
11. "I always wear a uniform and white shoes."	_____	_____
12. "The dental hygienist always develops her own X-rays."	_____	_____
13. "The receptionist opens the office and the dental assistant closes it in the evening."	_____	_____
14. "We never talk about other patients while working on someone else."	_____	_____
15. "We keep on schedule."	_____	_____
16. "We take responsibility for our own actions."	_____	_____

17. "The dentist never wears a uniform but all
    auxiliaries have to wear uniforms."   _____   _____
18. "On Saturdays we do not wear uniforms to
    the office."   _____   _____

SUMMARY

This chapter has dealt with the essential ingredients that make up a productive
and effective dental health team. A *dental health team* is a small group of
individuals with specific role delineations who are delivering preventive dental services on a regular basis. The four essential ingredients of a health team
are (1) communication, (2) interaction on a regular basis, (3) interdependence
of members, (4) recognition that team members are working toward common
goals. Factors influencing the team's effectiveness are structured variables
(e.g. size), independent or environmental variables (e.g., physical setting),
and the task-related variables (e.g., degree of difficulty). These are interrelated with intermediate variables, which in turn affect dependent variables.
All members of dental health teams have specific needs. The discussion
related these needs to Maslow's theory on human motivation—i.e, once the
physiological needs are met, team members will seek fulfillment of higher-
level needs (security, social, and self-actualization needs, for example). The
importance of developing specific cognitive and affective communication
skills cannot be overlooked by dental health professionals. A *communication
network* consists of a number of individuals who consistently interact with
one another on a daily basis in certain communication patterns. Such a network on a dental health team helps members better understand their own and
others' behavior. *System effects* are the influences of others on the behavior of
an individual team member's actions. The three concepts relating to communication networks discussed in this chapter are the total system, cliques,
and personal communication networks. Each type plays a part in the total
effectiveness of any working group. Conversations with health professionals
indicate that the level of cohesiveness within the working group is an important factor in team effectiveness. *Cohesiveness* refers to the ability of the team
to work together as one unit toward a common set of goals. Specific ways for a
dental health team to build cohesiveness require knowledge of the dynamics
of the team, including setting goals, paying close attention to leadership styles
and various roles undertaken by team members, cooperative team evaluation, and awareness of team norms. Knowing what the team is trying to
accomplish and where it is going is essential if any working group is to be productive and cohesive. Being conscious of the four leadership styles
(authoritative, consultive, democratic, and laissez-faire) that emerge for-

mally and informally within a group can benefit any team member. Roles undertaken by team members include task-related roles, maintenance roles, and individual roles. It is important for any team to periodically evaluate its goals, productivity, job satisfaction, and the quality of dental care it is providing. *Group norms* are the evolved nonverbal and verbal rules which influence the actions of team members. They are the habits that are acceptable in a dental office.

CHAPTER ACTIVITIES

1. Based on the four essential ingredients which help people work toward a common goal in a group, analyze a staff meeting or other small group according to each criterion.
2. Using your own school or a dental team with which you are familiar, draw a diagram of the organizational structure, including areas in which "cliques" exist.
3. Using the variables illustrated in Figure 9–1, describe an existing group according to the functions listed as factors that influence the effectiveness of a dental health team. You need not use a dental group for this exercise.
4. In a group of classmates or fellow staff members, discuss a common task or problem with which your group needs to deal. After doing so, and while the discussion is fresh in your mind, make a list of the cognitive and affective behavior skills enumerated in this chapter and identify the members of your group by putting their initials next to each skill that corresponds to their behavior in the group.
5. Using the same list of behavior skills, at the end of a day at school or in the clinic, write a one-sentence description of which skills you used and how you used them.
6. Using the descriptions of task roles, maintenance roles, and individual roles mentioned in this chapter, describe the roles taken by a small group of people with whom you live, work, or socialize regularly. (Some people take on several roles.)

REFERENCES

* Quoted by James I. Siress, senior consultant, Lawrence Leiter and Company, Management Consultants, Kansas City, Missouri.

1. For additional definitions of working teams, see Ernest G. Bormann and Nancy C. Bormann, *Effective Small Group Communication*, 2nd ed. (Minneapolis: Burgess, 1976), p. 44; Mark S. Zivan and Beverly G. Singleton, *A Manager's Guide to Human Behavior*, American Management Associations Extension In-

stitute (Education for Management Inc., 1971), pp. 19–20; John W. Keltner, "Interacting with Others: Face to Face in a Small Group," in *Interpersonal Speech Communication: Elements and Structures* (Belmont, Cal.: Wadsworth Publishing Company, Inc., 1970), pp. 289–315.

2. Zivan and Singleton, *A Manager's Guide to Human Behavior*, p. 20.

3. Zivan and Singleton, *A Manager's Guide*, pp. 28–30.

4. For additional information, see Ibid., pp. 28–30; also Jack R. Gibb, "Defensive Communication," *The Journal of Communication*, 11 (1961), 141–48; Bormann and Bormann, *Effective Small Group Communication*, pp. 43–70.

5. See Everett M. Rogers and Rekha Agarwala-Rogers, *Communication in Organizations* (New York: The Free Press, 1976), p. 108.

6. Ibid., pp. 111–12.

7. Ibid., pp. 108–48.

8. Ibid., pp. 113–15, 141–42.

9. See Bormann and Bormann, *Effective Small Group Communication*, pp. 70–72.

10. See John F. Cragan and David W. Wright, *Communication in Small Group Discussions* (St. Paul, Minn.: West Publishing Co., 1980), p. 73.

11. Bormann and Bormann, *Effective Small Group Communication*, p. 101.

12. Lee Thayer, "Communication and Organization Theory," in *Human Communication Theory: Original Essays*, Frank E. X. Dance, ed. (New York: Holt, Rinehart & Winston, 1967), p. 93.

13. The "gate keeper" role in the flow of information was described first by Kurt Lewin in "Frontiers in Group Dynamics: Channels of Group Life," *Human Relations* I (1947), 143–63.

14. Cragan and Wright, *Communication in Small Group Discussions*, p. 57, see also Bormann and Bormann, *Effective Small Group Communication*, pp. 56–58.

15. Ibid., p. 57.

Conflict Management and Problem Solving

10

What are the most effective ways to solve problems and manage the inevitable conflicts that occur within a dental health team? Finding an answer to this question is crucial to the team. The cooperation of all members is essential, if problems are to be resolved and serious conflicts avoided. But this is more easily said than done, as the following examples illustrate.

> Salary is the biggest conflict because money is the prime motivation for working.
>
> *A Registered Dental Hygienist*

> The doctor never made criticism in a constructive way.
>
> *A Registered Dental Hygienist*

> I always thought there was a barrier between hygienists and dental assistants. But when I started working, I really did not feel that way at all. I think it has a lot to do with personality. If you work with them, they will work with you.
>
> *A Certified Dental Assistant*

> The first dental hygienist we had in the office would only do dental hygiene. But the second hygienist would help me out anytime she could. It helped our efficiency. But the receptionist had no dental training and refused to try to learn; if she had learned, the entire office would have run more smoothly.
>
> *A Certified Dental Assistant*

200

Trust levels here are not very high.

A Registered Dental Hygienist

Conflicts will always occur among people who live, work, or play together regularly. Conflicts also occur among people who encounter each other just by chance. Conflicts are not unusual. In fact, they occur so often and in so many ways that we may not even identify them as such, either because they can easily be resolved or because we do not want to consider them conflicts. Conflict is something we often try to wish away, making believe it is not there. It seems to be a part of our social etiquette not to admit that such a state is possible, or perhaps it is our pride that makes us feel that any problem can be solved before it actually becomes a "conflict."

This chapter deals with conflicts and problem solving. Not all problems are conflicts. But all conflicts are problems. The question we need to ask each time there is a problem or a conflict is, "Do we want to resolve the conflict or solve the problem in a *constructive* or a *destructive* way?" We, the authors, state our bias at the outset—namely, that we believe that conflicts should be resolved in a constructive way and that problems should be solved creatively. Because problems need not be conflicts and because unsolved problems can, eventually, lead to conflicts, we will discuss problem solving first.

PROBLEM SOLVING

It is possible to distinguish between the concepts of problem solving and conflict resolution by observing whether or not those involved are cooperating or competing. Cooperation and consensus are important to problem solving. Creative problem solving can be done by following the following basic steps:[1]

1. State the problem.
2. Find facts and information about the problem.
3. Find ideas, brainstorm.
4. Find criteria to test ideas.
5. Find the solution.
6. Find acceptance for implementation.

STATE THE PROBLEM.   This step may not be as easy as it seems. If you select an issue that is not the actual problem, then all your efforts will lead to irrelevant "solutions" that will not be helpful. The way you state the problem is important, too. The Creative Problem Solving Institute suggests that a problem be stated in the form of a question allowing for many possibilities. To do this, begin the statement with the words, "In what ways might we . . . ?" The word "ways" allows for the possibility of many solutions; the word "might" opens us to the possibility of flexibility and creativity, unlike the word "should," which implies that there is a single correct solution; and the pronoun "we" lets everyone know that each person is involved and that this is not going to be a power play on the part of any one person or any clique in the group.

Find Facts.   State as many facts as you can which relate to the problem. It is good to have something to write on which everyone can see. If there are two people, a single piece of paper on a desk might be enough. If the group is larger, a chalkboard or sheets of newsprint secured to the wall with masking tape will help. Jot down everything factual that you and the group can think of. Be careful to avoid opinions here. Use data like numbers, names, dates.

Find Ideas; Brainstorm.   This stage is the most fun and it is one for which everyone should follow the rule of "deferred judgment." In this step it is necessary for all involved to assume that there are no wrong ideas. During this stage, everyone thinks of *any* idea that might work, no matter how wild or unworkable it might seem. All suggestions should be allowed without comment, without judgmental remarks like "Oh, we've tried that," or "That's silly," or "We've never done anything that way before." One suggestion might be to have everyone jot down ten ideas on a piece of paper, in short phrases, then share them all. As one person hears an idea it may trigger a similar idea that can be "piggy-backed" onto the first. A so-called "crazy" idea may trigger less crazy ideas if all ideas are allowed to flow freely. This allows creativity and flexibility and may produce several ideas which no one has considered before. Again, it is helpful to jot these down on paper or a board where all can see every idea. Get as many ideas—even those which seem alike but have subtle differences—as you can in the time you have.

Find Criteria to Test the Ideas.   Whereas the brainstorming stage suspends all judgments, during this stage specific criteria, or tests, are selected which apply to the problem at hand. Again, as with previous steps, consensus is important. Ask yourselves what factors will determine whether or not the ideas will work. If you have three days to find a solution, then one criterion would be "Time: 3 Days." Perhaps some of the information from the fact-finding stage, such as money, will be a criterion.

Find the Solution.   By consensus (not by vote), select five or six of the many ideas that have been gathered during the brainstorming stage. These should be selected from the total list, and should seem to the group to be possibilities that will now be tested by the application of the criteria from step 4. On a grid (see Figure 10–1), place the ideas in a vertical column, with the criteria running along the top in a horizontal row. Apply the criteria to each idea by rating each idea with each criterion, applying a number from 0 to 5 to each idea.

CRITERIA

IDEAS	TIME	COST	PERSONNEL	ETC.	ETC.	ETC.	TOTAL
Idea #1							
Idea #2							
Idea #3							
Idea #4							

Figure 10–1. Solution-finding chart.

Once you have applied numerical ratings to each of the ideas in each of the criteria columns, you are ready to find the solution. This simply requires addition. Find the sum of each horizontal line for each idea. The sum total will result in choice of the solution which you, by your own criteria, determine to be workable. Whichever idea has the highest total is visibly your solution. If you have two or three with very close scores, ask if there are other criteria that might be applied. Sometimes the group will have a "feel" for, or express a verbal consensus, that one is the best choice when there is a tie. Finding the solution by consensus does not assure that it will be the *only* solution. And, in the case of a solution that involves implementation by people other than yourselves, the next step becomes the real test.

FIND ACCEPTANCE FOR IMPLEMENTATION. If it is you individually, or a pair, or a group, that must put the solution to work, then the implementation step is your doing just that. Or delegation of responsibilities may be the way to implement it. However, if you are not the one or ones with the power to implement the solution, then you must persuade another party that you have a workable solution (see the section on persuasion in Chapter 8). That may be another problem in itself.

An Example of Problem Solving in a Dental Office

The authors were invited to sit in on a staff meeting of a suburban dental office to observe the communication behavior of the group. During the meeting, several problems arose which, through consensus, were dealt with to the satisfaction of the whole group. It was, in communication behavior, a "healthy group." Here is an actual problem that arose—one which, if not solved, eventually would have led to serious intrastaff conflicts which in turn would have seriously hindered the effective process of preventive dental care for the patients. Because the problem was dealt with through open communication at a staff meeting, interpersonal conflict was averted. We shall use this problem as an example of how the problem-solving process can be followed.

PROBLEM AS PRESENTED.   There is a temperature problem.

DENTAL ASSISTANT: Doctor, is there any way we can control the temperature in the office?

DENTIST: Ah! That is a real problem. It wasn't this bad last year, was it? What did we do last winter?

DENTAL HYGIENIST: The problem is that it gets so hot in the operatory in the summer, and then, in the winter too, it is miserable for me and the patients.

CDA: It's so bad sometimes the M.O.D. won't solidify.

PROBLEM RESTATED.   In what ways might we lower the temperature in the operatories?

FACTS

> Temperature controls are not located in this office.
>
> Building owner has installed a new heating and cooling system.
>
> Building manager controls the temperature.
>
> Temperature control is for the entire building.
>
> Anything over 75°F. in the winter is too hot.
>
> Every time the front door opens in winter, it lets cold air into the waiting area.
>
> The front door opens to the outside.
>
> The receptionist's area is an open area which includes the waiting room.
>
> The receptionist has windows that can be opened.
>
> The operatories have no windows.
>
> Heat makes everyone miserable.
>
> Heat melts the M.O.D.
>
> When heat melts the M.O.D., it has to be redone.
>
> Redoing M.O.D. makes the patient wait longer.

IDEAS

> Open the windows.
>
> Complain to the building manager.

Close the vents in the waiting room in the summer to force cooler air into the operatories.

Keep doors open in the operatories.

Sue the landlord for every M.O.D. melted.

Move to another building.

Get every tenant to sign a petition.

Buy fans for the operatories.

Don't pay the rent when it gets too hot.

Bring the landlord down to sit in a hot operatory for an hour.

Talk the RDH's husband into buying the building.

Get a new building manager.

Learn to suffer.

(Can you think of others?)

CRITERIA AND CRITERIA APPLICATION

SOLUTION.   Mathematically, "complaining to the building manager" was the best solution. This solution had been attempted before. However, the last time the dentist had complained, he did so in the form of a spoken request. The staff agreed that this time a complaint should be bolstered with a list of the reasons why temperature control should be taken seriously.

IMPLEMENTATION.   The dentist was the person who would make the complaint, since he, technically, was the lessee and the one who paid the bills. He volunteered to do this and the staff confirmed this, verbally and nonverbally, by consensus. The thought also occurred to one of the staff members that the dentist might consult with other lessees to see if a joint complaint might be more influential. As far as this staff was concerned, they had done all they could at that moment to solve the problem. This decision allowed the problem to remain at the problem-oriented stage and not to become an interpersonal conflict.

Figure 10–2. Criteria and criteria-application chart.

	Apply to All Rooms	Acceptable to Manager	Uniform Temperature	Cost Minimal	Total
1. Open windows	3	3	0	5	11
3. Close vents	3	5	0	5	13
8. Buy fans	3	5	0	0	8
2. Complain	5	2	5	5	17

CONFLICT

In Chapter 5, "Communication Choices," the guiding philosophy was that we do have choices about how we communicate. From our own self-concept and perception of others, we make choices that we think are appropriate to the situation. We can rarely control the other person's choices. Still, communication, by definition, involves several elements, including sending, receiving, and responding to information, one from the other(s). Because of this, communication is at once an *individual* act *and* an *interrelated* act. We make our own choices, but these depend on the *relationship* with the other person(s). Conflict, then, as a condition of communication, exists as a perception within us, because of a relationship we have with one or more other people.

Conflict generally exists when a problem cannot be solved cooperatively by the two or more people affected by the problem. It is generally resolved when communication choices occur in a productive way between all those people involved. Of course, it can result also in alienation and destruction, depending on the attitudes, values, goals, and communication choices of the participants. The authors believe that conflict should be resolved productively for all persons involved, without alienation or destruction. This value is reflected in the content of the remainder of this chapter.

A conflict situation exists, according to Joyce Hocker Frost and William Wilmot, when the following elements exist:[2]

1. An expressed struggle
2. Perceived incompatible goals
3. Perceived scarce rewards
4. Interdependence and independence

With these in mind, read the following description of a situation taken from an interview with a Registered Dental Hygienist. See how many of the four elements given above you can identify.

> I think the biggest problem in our office is that I do not agree with all the dentist's philosophies, but his dental assistants do. He has trained them himself. Then, here I come out of an accredited program with ideas and ethics which don't match his. For example, he thinks every cracked M.O.D. automatically should be crowned. I disagree. He knows our philosophies are not compatible, so he takes it out on me by making my patients wait 30 to 40 minutes before he checks them. Meanwhile, other patients are in the waiting room and I am constantly working into the noon hour.

First, this expressed conflict is a struggle between the RDH and apparently, everyone in the office who works directly with the dentist. But the central figures are the RDH and the dentist. Second, their "philosophies" which could be redefined as the goals of preventive dentistry, are different. In the same interview, this dental hygienist also revealed that the dentist believed it was important to give new patients a tour of the office but not important to offer instructions on preventive dental care. The RDH felt that time was wasted by the tour, time that could be better used in education—again, incompatible goals. Third, the RDH perceived scarce rewards, not in terms of salary but in terms of cooperation. Finally, because of their presence together on the same staff, there was both independence and interdependence—or as we prefer to label it, interrelatedness.

A second situation is explained by a Certified Dental Assistant who was the third person on the team in a small, private practice.

> In the practice where I worked, the dentist's mother-in-law was the receptionist. She only did bookwork. She would not pour up a study model, or take an X-ray, even though she knows how to do these things. All she would do would be to seat a patient in the operatory. Even though we needed her to assist in other ways, I did not feel free to discuss this with the dentist and I became frustrated because of the family ties.

This situation was perceived by the CDA as a conflict in which she felt as though she was powerless. Whether or not, in fact, she was indeed unable to change the situation to a more compatible one, is not the conflict. The conflict is the *perception* of the situation and her *choice* not to confront the dentist. Here, cultural and social values enter into the perceptions that influence the communication choice—in this case to remain silent and likely convey frustration in nonverbal ways.

Here is a third situation, as explained by a Registered Dental Hygienist who had just graduated from dental hygiene school and had begun her first practice in a small town with an established dentist. The practice was growing and the dentist hired both a Certified Dental Assistant and the RDH.

> For many years, Doctor _____ had one woman working for him. She was his receptionist and dental assistant. Then he hired a Certified Dental Assistant and me, a dental hygienist. We were hired at the same time. I was paid a salary higher than either of the assistants. The woman who had been with him for fifteen years complained about this to the dentist. The dentist was so glad to have a hygienist in his rural practice that he was not willing to lower my salary and wanted to support me as much as possible. The dentist resolved this conflict by raising the receptionist's salary to tide her emotions.

The dentist's action may not have resolved this conflict. In fact, it may have created a new one with the other dental assistant, if not immediately, then perhaps in the future. And the choice of the word "tide" used by the RDH to describe this situation may be prophetic. Tides go out and they come back. The dentist's willingness to give in when confronted may come back to haunt him if he is seen as an "easy touch." The younger assistant may want a raise, too. Also, the future ego conflicts that may result from the veteran assistant in conflict with the hygienist may create many spinoff conflicts.

Kinds of Conflict

What kinds of conflicts are there? In interviews with fifty dental auxilliaries, including dental hygienists and dental assistants working in dental clinics, private practice, and dental schools, we discovered that the most frequent conflicts deal with the following areas:

Money	This factor includes either salary inequities among staff members doing similar work or the lack of a standard scale, including overtime.
Personality and Ego	Problems in this category stem from attempts by auxiliaries to play "one-up" on the others, with winners and losers; or to form cliques, seek the dentist's favor over other auxiliaries; or to emphasize "superior" educational or years of experience, developing artificial hierarchies of importance.
Organizational Procedure	Conflicts in this area come from not knowing who makes decisions, not knowing how appointments are made and billings handled, confusion over scheduling, problems in obtaining assistance when needed, no clear communication lines.
Values and Philosophies Unclear Role Expectations	These involve attitudes about what is "best" or "right." Here, conflicts arise when auxiliaries are not clear about who does what for whom, and when. For example, when does an assistant help the receptionist answer the phone? Does the hygienist help the assistant clean instruments? If there are more than one dentist, who is the boss of whom? To whom do auxiliaries go with complaints and suggestions? What can a dentist expect from a Registered Dental Hygienist? What can a dentist expect from a Certified Dental Assistant with an accredited education compared with an assistant whom the dentist has trained?
Pseudo– Conflicts	In this case we have situations which appear to be conflicts but which are either misunderstandings or

limited views of possibilities. In logic, the latter is called an "either-or" fallacy, meaning that instead of only two choices, there are three or more. For example, "Either you water the plants or I will." A third choice is, of course, "You water the plants this week; I'll do it next week, and so on." Pseudo-conflicts can become real conflicts, however, if they are not identified early.

Defensive and Supportive Climates

Conflict exists, as we have said, when the persons involved are not able to cooperate in a problem-solving approach. And, although not all problems need to be solved by the six-step procedure described earlier in this chapter, problems solved by people who are cooperating with each other generally are solved by open communication and consensus. The communication environment has much to do with the way in which problems are either solved or turned into conflict. A now-famous description of defensive and supportive climates developed by Jack Gibb offers a list of contrasting attitudes that are easy to remember and applicable to almost any communication situation.[3] Knowledge of these climates is valuable in dealing with conflicts. Gibbs lists the following attitudes which determine the communication environment:

DEFENSIVE CLIMATES	SUPPORTIVE CLIMATES
1. Evaluation	1. Description
2. Control	2. Problem Orientation
3. Strategy	3. Spontaneity
4. Neutrality	4. Empathy
5. Superiority	5. Equality
6. Certainty	6. Provisionalism

Evaluation is judgmental, connotative, and subjective; *description*, on the other hand, is factual, denotative, and objective. *Control* occurs when one person tries to maneuver, manipulate, or persuade others to do things his or her way; in a *problem orientation* framework, however, each person focuses on the problem rather than on each other. *Strategy* involves planning ahead what to say in a discussion and thereby deciding on a unilateral solution; *spontaneity* allows ideas to arise between the participants in discussion in a common dialogue or group brainstorming session. *Neutrality* entails being uninvolved and disinterested, while *empathy*, as we have discussed elsewhere, is being aware of the others' needs and ideas through active listening and the ability to paraphrase with understanding what the others say. *Superiority* is the use of one's achievements, overtly, to show others that they are not as successful and competent; *equality*, however, involves a sense of mutual respect, one for the other, no matter how successful each is in his or her own life's work. *Certainty* is the "I know I'm right" attitude, and it closes off any other possibilities; *provisionalism*, in conflict resolution, is the openness to many possibilities.

Conflicts generally remain unresolved as long as parties to the conflict use defensive forms of communication. Problems come closer to being resolved under a supportive climate. In most interpersonal communication situations, when a person chooses defensive behavior, it is likely that the other person will also take on defensive behavior.

One case in which many of the defensive communication choices existed is one described in the following way by a Registered Dental Hygienist who worked on a dental staff headed by a female dentist.

> We really had a great team. There was the dentist, receptionist, another dental hygienist, dental assistant, and myself. We worked well together at first. In one day, for example, we saw five emergency patients. But the biggest problem was that the dentist never listened to us. Things got progressively worse. She (the dentist) became very judgmental. She needed to be in control of everything. Nothing was good enough unless she checked every detail herself. For instance, I was set up for an endodontic procedure and she felt that she needed to get out all the files and measure them. It made me wonder why I needed to set up this tray ahead of time if the doctor was going to check it. She did this kind of thing so often that it made me feel incompetent. None of us felt that the dentist trusted us. She would review all of my health histories in the presence of my patients. She never gave compliments and never thanked us for staying later—something we did regularly. Even though her number of patients was increasing, she was always saying, "I don't know how I'm going to pay you this week." It seemed like a game. Three months before I quit I tried to tell her what a great team she had, but that if she didn't listen to us and try to deal with the things that bothered us, it would all fall apart. Sure enough, when I left, the receptionist was the only one left.

In this case, the dentist created a defensive climate in which no problems were solved by discussion and, eventually, the problems escalated to conflict proportions and the staff quit. There was no attempt at conflict resolution on the part of the head of staff. This may have been due to a lack of organizational skills or the lack of communication training in the dentist's own professional education. It is truly a case in which most of the forms of defensive behavior existed.

The dentist was evaluative rather than descriptive in her way of dealing with salaries and in her nonverbal acts of checking the files and reviewing medical histories each time. She avoided dealing with problems as they were presented to her, thereby creating a situation in which dental auxiliaries learned that the only way out of a problem was to resign. If the dental hygienist was correct in her analysis that the dentist played games, this is both a form of control and a form of strategy. Her neutrality took the form of "Don't bother me with the facts," when she might have said, instead, "Tell me in what ways you think we could improve." Her attitude of superiority may derive from her hierarchy on the dental professional ladder. However, a sense of equality could have developed had the dentist respected the professional training and skill of the auxiliaries and allowed them to do their work with integrity—without rechecking every detail of their work. Because there apparently was never time taken for staff discussions or dialogue, provisionalism never could occur and the implied message of certainty grew strong as the dentist's way prevailed under all circumstances.

The concept of defensive and supportive behaviors can be helpful both to analyze a situation and to assist you in making communication choices that will cause conflicts to be constructively resolved.

COMMUNICATION EXERCISE 10-1

Which of the following comments or communication behaviors are examples of supportive and defensive climates in a dental office? Check the appropriate columns for each example, and in the third column specifically label the relevant attitude. Discuss your answers with your classmates or associates.

	SUPPORTIVE	DEFENSIVE	SPECIFIC ATTITUDE
1. "I think the reason people that have worked in this office leave is that they are not flexible."	_____	_____	_____
2. "I'm not going to let this girl think that she is going to run this office!"	_____	_____	_____
3. A patient comes into the dental hygienist's operatory with a book, sits down, proceeds to read, and does not look up when the hygienist begins the medical history review.	_____	_____	_____
4. The dentist says to a dental assistant, in front of a patient, "Do you think you did a good job?"	_____	_____	_____
5. At the end of a long day, the dental hygienist helps the dental assistant mount all the radiographs.	_____	_____	_____

(continued)

COMMUNICATION EXERCISE 10-1 *(Contd)*

6. The dentist says to his dental assistant, "I certainly could not manage without you."   _____ _____ _____

7. "If it is more convenient for you to have your appointment on another day, I will check our schedule and call you back in a few minutes."   _____ _____ _____

8. "It isn't my job to do that!"   _____ _____ _____

9. "I had been trying to get this particular patient into the office and he would always cancel or never show. This happened at least three or four times. Then one day, he walked into the office to get his teeth cleaned. The dentist said to work him into the schedule. It threw my schedule off an hour or more, and I had patients waiting."   _____ _____ _____

RESOLVING CONFLICT

Let us assume that a situation exists in which conflict exists between you and another dental auxilliary on the same dental team. You decide that you will either be able to resolve the conflict or you will have to leave and seek work elsewhere. What are some ways to work toward resolution?

1. *Identify the nature of the conflict.* Who is involved? What are the stated issues? Are all the elements of conflict present or is it, as you look closer, a pseudo-conflict based on misunderstanding or false conclusions? What is your role in the conflict? Know whether or not you are contributing to the intensity of the situation by verbal or nonverbal messages. How long has the problem existed? Who is most affected by the conflict and who would benefit most from its resolution? Would anyone benefit if the conflict intensified? Some people play games which develop conflict to force others to play by their win–lose rules. Who has power and knows it? Who feels weak or powerless? If you can list short answers to these questions you will begin to understand the nature of the conflict.

2. *Analyze the communication environment.* Is the climate supportive or defensive? Who talks with whom in a cooperative way? What kind of communication behavior do you observe, both in yourself and in others? Is there congruence between the words spoken and the nonverbal forms of com-

munication? If words denote calm objectivity but the rate and pitch of the voice are rapid and shrill, it may connote excited subjectivity. What do non-vocal–nonverbal forms of communication behavior tell you? Things like eye contact, turning toward or away from one who is talking, looking busy or bored, heavy sighs, unusual silence for long periods of time, and so forth may help you understand your own role in the conflict as well as who is siding with whom.

What is the content of the messages you hear and see? In general, you can study the content of messages and find that people are sending messages in any of the categories in Figure 10–3. By locating the conflict within some appropriate category you are able to focus on and aim your resolution at the appropriate target.

Also, in the communication environment, be aware of the networks with which you are working. You are a part of it, remember! What, if any, are the established hierarchies? How are problems usually solved? Is there an authoritarian, democratic, or laissez-faire system of decision making? Usually, there are unwritten rules about lines of communication and when and where different topics are most appropriately discussed.

3. *Deal with specific goals.* Once you have a picture of the nature of the conflict and the communication environment, you can begin to do this. You need to make some preliminary decisions yourself. We have already decided, for this discussion, that you do not want to let the problem exist without doing something about it. Let's assume, further, that you really want to resolve the problem rather than quitting your job. In making this assumption we have decided that your *goal* is to remain working as a productive member of this particular dental team. Making this goal decision is the step you need to take after analyzing the conflict and the communication situation. The com-

Figure 10–3. Message-sending categories.

CONTENT	ABOUT SELF	ABOUT OTHER INDIVIDUALS	ABOUT WHOLE GROUP	ABOUT TASK OR OBJECTIVES	ABOUT VALUES, PHILOSOPHIES OR GOALS
FACTUAL (Description)					
ANALYTICAL (Interpretation)					
JUDGMENTAL (Evaluation)					
EMOTIONAL (Expression of feelings)					

munication environment may be too "polluted," however, and you may not choose to wade through the complexity of the situation. Without outside third-party negotiation or arbitration, you may choose to quit. But let's say that your goal is to remain on the job and to work toward strengthening the existing preventive dental-care team.

4. *Decide on some specific objectives.* Objectives are those elements of the long-range goals which are specific, observable, identifiable. These are the actual things you can work toward immediately. Objectives deal with the issues that often cause problems, and that can develop into conflicts. In problem solving, it is the "statement of the problem" which is your objective, as we described earlier in this chapter. In conflict, you might try wording the objective in the same open-ended way you used in stating the problem. Instead of saying, "My objective is to get the receptionist to make appointments that correspond to a realistic workload and talk with me about cancellations," you can word it like this: "In what ways might we (the receptionist and you, and perhaps others on the staff) work out a realistic appointment schedule with regular communication about adjustments?" Or, another objective statement might go like this: "By the end of this week, I will have talked with the dentist and the receptionist, together, to develop a daily system of appointment checks." The objective, therefore, should

   a. Be stated in a way that is open to more than one possible solution
   b. Be inclusive of all parties affected
   c. Involve an observable behavioral change, stated clearly and concisely

Each of these is important. By being *open* to more than one way to resolve a conflict, you are making a choice about your own communication behavior—you are choosing to be what Gibb calls "supportive" or, in other words, choosing to give credibility to others' ideas, to respect their opinions and integrity, and to encourage openness on their part. To avoid this would be to create a defensive climate, one in which trust levels are low, debate may occur with a win–lose conclusion; ultimately a destructive climate could exist. By being *inclusive* you are making a choice to involve every affected party in the decision-making process. Because each one is involved, each person is more apt to be satisfied with the solution if he or she has an active part in the discussion. This is one of the basic conditions by which people are likely to change behavior. Their participation is perhaps just as important as winning their position, because of the assumption that they are important enough to be considered. If you choose not to be inclusive, to ignore someone or to purposely keep someone out of a discussion that directly affects them, alienation and not conflict resolution will be the result. If your overall goal is to have a cooperative, cohesive team, alienation is destructive to the wholeness you are seeking. Unilateral decisions (such as a dentist making a decision about pay raises without consulting everyone affected) usually are not as satisfactory in the long run as is consensus among the people who are party to the conflict.

Finally, stating objectives which include specific *behavioral change* will keep you on target. You will know when the conflict is resolved and will not prolong the situation longer than necessary. You can agree upon the results and stop the conflict. Otherwise, you might keep the conflict flickering for days without resolving it. Anything that prolongs unnecessary conflict on a dental team will eventually be felt by patients and have a negative effect on the practice itself.

5. *Decide on the method to achieve the objectives.* It is best, as we have already stated, to request that everyone who is involved in the conflict become involved in the resolution. Ask for a time to talk about just this problem. A special staff meeting or a few minutes set aside for a one-on-one talk in the privacy of an office with the door closed might be best. One dentist we know was flabbergasted one day when a dental assistant came into the operatory where he was with a patient and verbally let out her frustrations. His style was to deal with problems in his own office privately with his staff, not in the presence of patients. Eventually, this particular assistant lost her job because of this kind of insensitivity to appropriate times and places to deal with problems.

If, because the conflict has caused a strain in interpersonal relations, you do not feel able to confront the other person or persons directly, seek a third party as an intermediary. In labor relations, this person is called a negotiator. In such a situation the third party should not be a party to the conflict, but should be skilled in empathetic listening. Whether or not an outsider is involved, all staff persons involved still must be a part of the process. The third party listens to each and paraphrases back to each what he or she has heard in order to clarify the central issues. The negotiator (and this may be you if the conflict does not involve you directly but does exist in your office) may ask to talk privately, one at a time, with each side. During such discussions, the negotiator can ask for points on which each side is willing to make a compromise. If a problem has reached conflict proportions, there generally are two sides to the issue and compromise is almost always necessary to resolve the conflict.

Whether or not you need a negotiator, the key communication strategy here is to *involve every affected person in the process.*

Let everyone *state the issue* as they perceive it. If you do this, you may quickly discover how close to or how far apart you are from a resolution.

When everyone has stated his or her point of view, immediately acknowledge *points of agreement* that may arise. Starting with some points on which both sides agree leads toward common ground and may relieve some unnecessary tension.

Set a few rules everyone can live with. Try to set a time limit that is realistic for all of you to try to reach a resolution. Do your best to stick to this time, but avoid decisions that are too easy and superficial just to meet the time limit. Also, try to agree to *deal with the issue* and not with personal feelings about each other, if indeed the conflict is not over personalities. In the example given earlier of the assistant having a conflict with the tasks *not* done by the dentist's receptionist/mother-in-law, it would be best to deal with the tasks, and not the relationship problem.

Be an active listener and be willing to give descriptive feedback. Instead of planning what you are going to say next while your opponent is talking, pay attention to what is being said, and visibly show that you are hopeful that you will hear something that will be acceptable to you.

If your conflict is one involving personalities, egos, or other issues that are primarily subjective and not task- or job-related, you must make a choice about how *you* will behave, no matter what the other person's communication choices are. We suggest being *empathetic, open-minded, provisional, hopeful, descriptive, honest,* and willing to *treat the other person as valuable and important.* These patterns of behavior will not guarantee a resolution. The other person is free to behave any way he or she may choose. However, the power of *feedback* in the communication process (Chapter 2) is more important in conflict situations than are either persuasion or aggression. The distinction between assertiveness and aggression is a fine line. A person who is assertive may be *perceived* as being aggressive. Such perception will likely lead to a defensive posture by the other person. Once a defensive climate is established, it is difficult to overcome.

Finally, whatever power hierarchy may exist between you and the other party is best put aside during conflict resolution in an attempt to *see each other as equals.* If you are a subordinate on a dental team, there may be little you can do to influence this unless you can discuss the issue, after work, away from the dental environment. If you are in a higher professional category than the other person in the conflict it will be easier for you to choose this option.

COMMUNICATION EXERCISE 10-2

Below is the situation that appeared on page 206. Work through this exercise, pretending that you are the dental hygienist and using the five steps to resolve a conflict.

I think the biggest problem in our office is that I do not agree with all the dentist's philosophies, but his dental assistants do. He has trained them himself. Then, here I come out of an accredited program with ideas and ethics which don't match his. For example, he thinks every cracked M.O.D. automatically should be crowned. I disagree. He knows our philosophies are not compatible so he takes it out on me by making my patients wait 30 to 40 minutes before he checks them. Meanwhile, other patients are in the waiting room and I am constantly working into the noon hour. [In the same interview, this dental hygienist also revealed that the dentist believed it was important to give new patients a tour of the office but not important to offer instructions on preventive dental care.]

IDENTIFY THE NATURE OF THE CONFLICT. (These were given on page 208 of this text.)

1. Struggle between RDH and everyone in office who works directly with the dentist
2. Goals and philosophies of RDH and the dentist different
3. Scarce rewards
4. Interrelatedness

ANALYZE THE COMMUNICATION ENVIRONMENT

1. Is it supportive or defensive? (Underline the most appropriate.)
2. Give an example of a specific defensive climate behavior in this situation.
3. What nonverbal communication behaviors are displayed by the dentist in this situation?
4. What is the content of the message from the RDH?

DEAL WITH THE SPECIFIC GOALS

1. If you are the RDH, what will you chose as your goal? Will you quit, remain on the job and just exist, or remain on the job and work toward conflict resolution? If not any of these, what are other options?

SPECIFIC OBJECTIVES

1. If you are the RDH in this situation, what specific objectives will you pursue during the next few days?
   a.
   b.
   c.

DECIDE ON THE METHOD

1. How will you achieve your objectives if you are the RDH in this dental office?
   a.
   b.
   c.
   d.
   e.

COMMUNICATION EXERCISE 10-3

Below is an excerpt from a conversation with a Certified Dental Assistant. Using the five steps to resolve a conflict, pretend you are the dental assistant in this dental office. With another person,

1. Discuss the nature of the conflict
2. Analyze the communication environment
3. Determine specific goals
4. Determine specific objectives
5. Decide on your method of resolution

Conversation with CDA:

> The office I worked in had the dentist, two full-time dental assistants, a receptionist, and dental hygienist. The one dental assistant would not answer the telephone. I suggested to her that she should learn more about the front desk, because I believe the relationship between the dental assistant and the receptionist is so important in an office. Knowing about recall appointments and that it takes 45 minutes for a crown preparation helps me understand the importance of a receptionist job. It discouraged me that the other dental assistant would not try to learn. All she wanted to do was dental assisting. She would always say to me, "We don't have to do that. They didn't ask us to do that." I just believe that being able to answer the phone and make appointments if the receptionist is on an errand to the bank or dental laboratory is very important. The receptionist always would help us out in the back operatories when we needed assistance. I finally said to the other dental assistant that we needed more help out at the front desk. But her reply was, "It isn't my job to do that."

These steps can help you begin to work toward a resolution to conflict. If you discover that during the discussion there develops a cooperative rather than a competitive mood among members of the discussion, you may wish to move to the problem-solving process described earlier in this chapter.

SUMMARY

This chapter has presented two related topics, problem-solving and conflict resolution, as they relate to the work of dental auxiliaries with other members of the dental team. The six-step approach to creative problem-solving involves (1) stating the problem, (2) finding the facts, (3) finding ideas, (4) selecting the criteria, (5) finding the solution, and (6) finding acceptance for implementation. Problem-solving and conflict resolution can be distinguished in terms of the willingness of everyone to work cooperatively on a problem. There are many types of conflict situations, all of which include the following elements: (1) an expressed struggle, (2) perceived incompatible goals, (3) perceived scarce rewards, and (4) interdependence and independence. Six of the predominant issues which can lead to conflict among dental professionals concern money, personality and ego, organizational procedure, values and philosophies, unclear role expectations, and pseudo-conflicts. There are six contrasting attitudes involved in supportive and defensive communication which influence conflict climates: evaluation/description, control/problem orientation, strategy/spontaneity, neutrality/empathy, superiority/equality, and certainty/provisionalism.

Finally, the five stages of conflict resolution involve (1) identifying the nature of the conflict, (2) analysis of the communication environment, (3) dealing with specific goals, (4) deciding on specific objectives, stated in ways that are open to more than one solution and inclusive of all people involved and observable behavioral change, and (5) deciding on a method that will achieve the objectives, involving everyone in the process. Under difficult circumstances, a third party might be involved as a negotiator or arbitrator.

The authors have discovered in interviews with dental professionals that the subject matter of this chapter may well be the most vital to an effective dental team, together with the technical skills learned in clinical education. This has been a chapter, however, which depends on your fundamental knowledge of all preceding chapters. This culminating chapter may help you realize the importance of this textbook—namely, the significance of knowing effective communication skills for the practice of your chosen profession.

CHAPTER ACTIVITIES

1. Together with two other students or associates, or by yourself, select a problem that you would like to solve. Using the six steps listed in this chapter, work through your problem in the creative problem-solving process. Use a chalkboard or large sheets of newsprint taped on walls in the room so that everyone can clearly see the information given in each step. When you are finished, name the people who would need to implement this solution and describe briefly any barriers that might occur in the "acceptance" stage.

2. Interview a practicing dental auxiliary, asking for a description of any staff conflict that has occurred recently. See how many of the Frost and Wilmot elements of conflict exist.

3. Think of the last time you were in conflict with another person. Using the six contrasting types of supportive and defensive behaviors described in

this chapter, write a one-sentence description of examples of any of these behaviors which applied to your situation.

4. Attend a staff meeting and observe whether there are either problems or conflicts being discussed. If there are problems, analyze how they are solved, using the six-step process discussed in this chapter. If there are conflicts, use Figure 10–1 in this chapter to analyze the categories of communication.

REFERENCES

1. Adapted from the Creative Problem Solving Workshop at the Creative Problem Solving Institute, State University College at Buffalo, N.Y., June 16–June 21, 1973. See also George R. Eckstein, "Pleasure for the Creative Mind," in *The Creative Process*, Angelo M. Biondi, ed. (Buffalo: The Creative Education Foundation, Inc., D.O.K. Publishers, Inc., 1972), pp. 1–4.
2. Joyce Hocker Frost and William W. Wilmot, *Interpersonal Conflict* (Dubuque, Ia.: W. C. Brown, 1978), pp. 3–15.
3. Jack R. Gibb, "Defensive Communication," *The Journal of Communication*, 11: (1961), 141–148. Used with permission.

BIBLIOGRAPHY

BORMANN, ERNEST G. and BORMANN, NANCY C., *Effective Small Group Communication*, 2nd ed. Minneapolis: Burgess, 1976.

CIVIKLY, JEAN M., ed., *Messages, a Reader in Human Communication*. New York: Random House, 1974.

CRAGAN, JOHN F., and WRIGHT, DAVID W., *Communication in Small Group Discussions*. St. Paul, Minn.: West Publishing Company, 1980.

FROST (WILMOT), HOCKER, JOYCE, and WILMOT, WILLIAM W. *Interpersonal Conflict*. Dubuque, Ia.: Wm. C. Brown, 1978.

GIBB, JACK R., "Defensive Communication," *The Journal of Communication*, 11 (1961), 141–48.

KELTNER, JOHN W., "Communication and the Labor Management Mediation Process: Some Aspects and Hypothesis," *The Journal of Communication*, XV (June 1965).

KELTNER, JOHN W. "Interacting with Others: Face to Face in a Small Group," *Interpersonal Speech Communication: Elements and Structures*. Belmont, Cal.: Wadsworth, 1970, 289–315.

LEWIN, KURT, "Frontiers in Group Dynamics: Channels of Group Life," *Human Relations* I (1947), 143–53.

ROGERS, EVERETT M., and AGARWALA-ROGERS, REKHA, *Communication in Organizations*. New York: The Free Press, 1976.

RUBIN, IRWIN M., PLOVRICH, MARK S., and FRY, RONALD E., *Improving the Coordination of Care: A Program for Health Team Development.* Cambridge, Mass: Ballinger, 1975.

THAYER, LEE, "Communication and Organization Theory," in *Human Communication Theory: Original Essays,* Frank E. X. Dance, ed. New York: Holt, Rinehart & Winston, 1967.

VERDERBER, RUDOLPH I., and VERDERBER, KATHLEEN S., *Inter-Act: Using Interpersonal Communication Skills,* 2nd ed. Belmont, Cal.: Wadsworth, 1980.

ZIVAN, MARK S., and SINGLETON, BEVERLY G., *A Manager's Guide to Human Behavior,* American Management Associations Extension Institute. Education for Management, Inc., 1977.

GLOSSARY

Acceptance: Occurs, in dialogue, when the initial message is seen as valid and is agreed upon by both parties.

Action: The final step in dialogue. Each person takes common action on the matter about which they have agreed and which they have internalized.

Articulation: Formation of vocal sounds by the tongue, teeth, and lips into specific speech sounds.

Assertiveness: Type of behavior in which one person transmits a message to another, honestly and directly, without fear of what the other might feel or expect in return, while respecting the uniqueness of the other person.

Authoritarian Communication: Occurs when one person perceives herself or himself as having more power or expertise than another and consequently makes demands, issues orders, or makes assumptions about the behavior of the other person.

Channel: The medium or media by which the message is sent (e.g., light waves allow facial expressions to be seen; a dress style carries the message of the wearer's personality).

Cliques: A subsystem in which members interact more frequently with one another than with other members on a team.

Cohesiveness: The ability of the team to work together as one unit toward a common goal.

Communication: The process of sharing messages.

Communication Network: Consists of a number of individuals who persistently interact with one another on a daily basis in certain communication patterns.

Conflict: A condition of disagreement which exists as a perception of a relationship, resulting in an inability to solve problems cooperatively.

Connotative Meaning: The meaning implied by a word.

Contact: In dialogue, the sensory reception of one's message transmission by another person.

Decoding: The stage in communication at which the message that has been sent is selectively interpreted for meaning. Parts of the original message may be filtered out by physical or mental interference.

Deductive Learning: Occurs when a student is told what he or she needs to know or how to perform a particular skill by a teacher who provides the information; the student is a receiver of information.

Denotative Meaning: The literal or dictionary meaning of a word.

Dental Health Team: A small group of individuals who have specific role delineations and are delivering preventive dental services on a regular basis.

Destination: The final stage in the message-sending process; e.g., the person who receives the message.

Dialogue: Two parties communicating together by completing the seven steps of interpersonal communication which include: transmission, contact, feedback, understanding, acceptance, internalization, action.

Emotion: A human trait that sets the mood, places emphasis, and reinforces the value of message content. Also called *pathos.*

Encoding: The process of putting the message into an intelligible code, such as language or other symbols that carry meaning.

Feedback: The response or message returned to the original sender of the message by the receiver, providing the sender with knowledge of results about the initial, encoded message.

Field of Experience: The realm of human experiences which influence each individual's values, perceptions, and communication behavior. When fields of experience overlap, communication is usually improved.

Group Dynamics: The communication behavior of all individuals in a group as it affects both the group as a whole and individual members.

Group Norm: Nonverbal and verbal rules which influence the actions of the team members.

Inductive Learning: Occurs when the student discovers by experiencing what should be learned. A teacher may design and guide the process of learning, but the student seeks out the information and skills.

Intercultural Communication: Communication between members of two or more identifiable communities with different cultural backgrounds.

Internalization: Occurs when the thoughts and messages of one person in a dialogue become a part of the thoughts and messages of the second person in an interpersonal transaction. Each "owns" the other's ideas.

Interpersonal Communication: Occurs when two people send and receive messages to and from one another. Also called *Dyadic Communication.*

Intrapersonal Communication: The sending and receiving of messages within one person both mentally and physiologically.

Learning: The acquisition of knowledge or of a skill.

Maintenance Roles: Those roles which keep the team functioning no matter what the task may be.

Mass Communication: Communication with a diverse, dispersed audience that is too large to be in one place at one time, and is unseen by the sender. Usually uses electronic or print media.

Motivation: That which stimulates or compels an individual, internally, to act.

Nonverbal–Nonvocal Communication: The use of behavior other than speech, writing, or vocal sound to send messages and the corresponding use of the senses of touch, taste, and smell in communication, e.g., the use of bodily movement and facial expression; also called kinesics. The placement of persons in relation to each other; also called proxemics. Touch or tactile communication.

Perception: The process by which a person sorts the sensory stimuli from past experiences into assumptions and impressions that are transferrable to present and future situations, helping him or her to make communication choices to fit the occasion.

Personal Communication Networks: The patterns of interaction that individual members of a group establish with and among themselves.

Persuasion: The external influences that compel an individual to act.

Private Agenda: Ideas, plans, and any general thoughts in one's mind that distract a listener from what the speaker is saying.

Pronunciation: The manner of articulation which causes the word sounds to be understood in a particular language region.

Public Communication: The sharing of messages with a large group of people, as in speeches given to audiences and lectures given in educational settings.

Reason: The logical arrangement of ideas in words and sentences to explain and to persuade. Also called *Logos.*

Selective Listening: Listening for only isolated information, taking words and meanings out of their intended encoded context.

Selective Perception: Allowing oneself to be aware of only those aspects of another person's verbal and nonverbal behavior which fits one's own stereotype or preconceived view of that person.

Small-group Communication: Communication within a group of three to (about) seventeen persons, who meet for different reasons, including information sharing, decision making, problem solving, therapy, and social entertainment.

Source: Where the message begins and to which feedback may return.

Stereotyping: Having fixed assumptions and expectations of people.

Style: How an individual selects words and arranges them in a particular way using grammar and syntax to form meaningful sentences and verbal expressions.

System Effects: The influence of a group process on the behavior of an individual team member's actions.

Task Roles: Activities performed by individual team members to get their job done.

Transmission: The sending of messages from one person to another.

Total System Communication Network: The communication patterns that develop among all the members of a particular team.

Understanding: The comprehension of another's message, the fourth stage in dialogue.

Verbal Communication: The use of words, in speaking or writing, to convey a message.

Vocal Communication: The use of sounds, such as the pitch and tone of voice, the volume of sound, and the articulation of sound into speech, to convey a message.

Index

A

Acceptance, 19
Accuracy in verbal communication, 82
Action, 20
Agarwala-Rogers, Rekha, 178
Age, perceptions and, 54
Appropriateness:
    of nonverbal–nonvocal communication, 102
    of verbal communication, 84
    of vocal communication, 87–89
Approval of others, 49
Ariando, A. A., 148
Aristotle, 77
Articulation, 85–87
Assertiveness, 21–22
Assigned roles, 66–67
Attitudes, 30, 31, 55–61
    change in, 151–53
Authoritativeness, 21–22
    leadership and, 186

B

Beavin, Janet Helmick, 29, 69
Behavioral change, 151–53

Behavior management, 143–44
Berger, Charles R., 73
Berlo, David, 30, 37
Body movements (kinesics), 35, 90–93
Brainstorming, 202
Brooks, William O., 43
Buber, Martin, 76, 89

C

Calabrese, Richard J., 73
Career choice, 50
Central nervous system, 14
Certainty, 209, 210
Chosen roles, 67–69
Clarifying response, 127
Cliques, 177, 178–79
Closed questions, 126
Closure, 129
Code, professional, 58–59
Cognitive behavior skills, 175
Cohesiveness, 179–83
Communication:
    definition of, 3, 13
    emphasis on, 1–3
    factors affecting, 30–31

Communication (*Contd.*)
   intercultural, 24–25
   interpersonal, 16–22, 117–20
   intrapersonal, 14–15
   mass, 25–26
   models for dental auxiliaries, 32–36
   nonverbal-nonvocal (*see* Nonverbal-
      nonvocal communication)
   organizational (*see* Dental health
      team)
   personal aspects of, 77–79
   public, 22–24
   Schramm model of, 28–32, 35
   small-group, 22
   tactile, 35, 94, 96
   telephone, 88, 118
   types of, 13–26
   verbal (*see* Verbal communication)
   vocal (*see* Vocal communication)
   (*see also* Perceptions; Roles)
Communication networks, 176–79
Communication skills, 30
Competency, 144–45
Conflict, dental health team and, 6–7,
      200–201, 206–18
Conflict resolution, 6–7
Congruency, 175
Connotative meaning, 79, 82, 135, 156
Consultative leadership, 186
Contact, 18
Control, 209, 211
Creative Problem Solving Institute, 200
Cultural perceptions, 59–60
Cultural roles, 64

D

Decoding, 29, 32, 76
Deductive approach, 147
Defensive climates, 209–11
Defensiveness, 134–35
Deferred judgment, 202
Democratic leadership, 186
Denotative meaning, 79, 82, 135, 136
Dental environment, 4, 114–17
Dental health team, 167–221
   basic ingredients for successful, 169
   cohesiveness and, 179–83
   communication networks, 176–79
   conflict, 6–7, 200–201, 206–18
   definition of, 168–69
   evaluation, 194–95

Dental health team (*Contd.*)
   evolution of, 173–76
   factors influencing effectiveness of,
      169–72
   group norms, 195–97
   leadership styles, 184–87
   needs of members of, 172–73
   problem solving, 200–205
   roles, 174, 187–94
Description, 209
Destination, 29
Dialogue, 20
Distance, 93–95
Dress, 99–102
Dworkin, Samuel F., 152
Dyadic communication, 16–22, 117–20

E

Edney, J. J., 94
Education, 32–36 (*see also* Learning
     theories)
Emmert, Phillip, 43
Emotions, 32–36, 77, 78
   attachment to roles, 66
   perceptions and, 55–60
Empathy, 152, 175–76, 209
Encoding, 29–31, 76
Environment, 4, 32–36, 114–17
Equality, 209, 210, 211
Equipment, 96–97
Evaluation, 209
   of dental health team, 194–95
   of patient, 119–20
   role, 66–67, 134
Experience, 32–36
Eye contact, 93, 94, 118, 135

F

Facial expressions, 90–93
Family roles, 65
Fear:
   as motivator, 150–51
   reduction, 145–46
Feedback, 18–19, 32, 35, 69–72, 216
Feshbach, H., 150, 151, 156
Festinger, Leon, 151
First impressions, 50–51, 111–21
   interpersonal encounter, 117–20
   physical environment, 114–17
Flexibility, 175

Frame of reference, 174
Frost, Joyce Hocker, 206
Fully Human, Fully Alive (Powell), 46,
    48

G

Gagné, Robert, 145
Gender, perceptions and, 54
Genuineness, 175
Gibb, Jack, 209, 214
Goals, 213–14
    establishing team, 184
    of interviews, 124
Grooming, 99–102
Group consensus, 151–52
Group Dynamics movement, 152
Group norms, 195–97
Group organization, 187

H

Hall, Edward T., 99
Hearing, 35
Hein, Eleanor, 31
Helm, Sharon, 21
Hierarchy of human needs, 150, 173

I

Identity, 4–5, 49
Illustration, 83
Impatience, 135
Individual roles, 193–94
Inductive approach, 147, 148–49
Initiative, 175
Intercultural communication, 24–25
Internalization, 19–20
Interpersonal communication, 16–22,
    117–20
Interpretative response, 126–27
Interviews, 88–89, 123–33, 155
    goals of, 124
    techniques for, 124–29
    typical, 130–33
Intrapersonal communication, 14–15

J

Jackson, Don D., 29, 69
Janis, I. L., 150, 151, 156

K

Katz, Daniel, 11
Kegeles, S. Stephan, 152–53
Knowledge level, 30, 31

L

Lackey, Arlen D., 72
Laissez-faire leadership, 186, 187
Leadership, 2
Leadership styles, 2, 184–87
Leading questions, 127–28
Learning theories, 141–49
    behavior management, 143–44
    competency, 144–45
    deductive approach, 147
    definition of learning, 142
    examples of, 157–59
    fear reduction, 145–46
    inductive approach, 147, 148–49
    satisfying needs, 142–43
Lewin, Kurt, 143, 151
Listening, 2, 123, 133–36, 155
    guidelines for good, 135–36
    problems in, 133–35
Love, 48

M

Maintenance roles, 192–93
Maslow, Abraham, 150, 173
Mass communication, 25–26
Meaning, 79, 81
Motivation, 141–42, 148, 150–54
    attitude and behavior change,
        151–53
    examples of, 157–59
    fear and, 150–51
    hierarchy of needs, 150, 173
Mowrer, O. H., 145–46

N

National Opinion Research Center, 71
Needs:
    hierarchy of, 150, 173
    satisfying, 142–43
Negative feedback, 69
Negative perceptions, 52
Neutrality, 209, 211
Neutral perceptions, 52

Nonverbal-nonvocal communication,
    18, 89–102, 128, 135
  appropriateness, 102
  body movements, 90–93
  definition of, 78
  distance, 93–95
  dress and grooming, 99–102
  equipment, 96–97
  facial expressions, 90–93
  odor, 97–98
  status, 98–99
  time, 99
  touch, 94, 96

O

Objective description, 82–83
Objectives, 214–15
Odor, 97–98
Open-ended questions, 124, 126
Openness, 175
Operant conditioning, 143–44, 148
Operatory, 115–17
Others, perception of, 50–52, 173–74

P

Paraphrasing, 128–29
Patient feedback, 69–72
Perceptions, 35–36, 43–62, 153
  changed, 43
  cultural, 59–60
  definition of, 43–45
  factors affecting, 53–60
  of others, 50–52, 173–74
  of patients, 71–72
  selective, 51–52
  of self, 45–50, 173–74
  types of, 52
Personal appearance, 99–102
Personal communication networks,
    177–78
Personal perception choices, 52–60
Persuasion, 141–42, 154–57
  examples of, 157–59
Phillips, J. Donald, 165
Positive feedback, 69
Positive perceptions, 62
Powell, John, 46, 48
Pride, 176
Private agenda planning, 133, 136
Probing responses, 127

Problem orientation, 209
Problem solving, 6–7
  dental health team and, 200–205
Pronunciation, 85–87
Provisionalism, 209, 210, 211
Psychological process, 14
Public communication, 22–24

R

Race, perceptions and, 54
Rate of speech, 86
Reason, 77–78
Receptionist, role of, 117, 119
Reid, Clyde, 16, 26
Religion, perceptions and, 54–55
Repetition, 126
Responses, 35–36
  clarifying, 127
  evaluating patients', 136–38
  interpretative, 126–27
  probing, 127
Responsibility, 175
Rogers, Carl, 56, 152
Rogers, Everett M., 178
Rokeach, Milton, 57
Role(s), 60, 63–75
  ambiguity, 188–89
  assigned, 66–67
  chosen, 67–69
  cultural, 64
  definition of, 63–64
  dental context, 72–73
  dental health team and, 174, 187–94
  emotional attachment to, 66
  evaluation, 189–94
  expectations, 66–67, 134
  family, 65
  individual, 193–94
  maintenance, 192–93
  models, 49–50
  patient feedback, 69–72
  playing, 49, 102
  social, 64
  task, 190–91
  work, 65–66
Role-taking, 49, 67–69

S

Scandura, Joseph, 145
Schramm, Wilbur, 28–32, 35, 37

Selective listening, 134
Selective perception, 51–52
Self-acceptance, 48–50
Self-concept, 5, 119
Self-fulfilling prophecy, 45
Self-inventory, 46–48
Self-perception, 49–50, 173–74
Self-respect, 175
Senses, 14, 15, 35
Signal, 29
Silent arguing, 134–35
Skinner, B. F., 143, 148
Small-group communication, 22
Smell, 35
Socialization messages, 56
Social roles, 64
Societal demands, 60
Sound production, 85
Source, 28–29, 31
Speech (see Vocal communication)
Spontaneity, 209
Status, 98–99
Stereotypes, 119, 134
Strategy, 209, 211
Style of verbal communication, 81–84
Summarizing, 128
Superiority, 209, 211
Supportive climates, 209–11
System effects, 176

T

Tactile communication, 35, 94, 96
Task roles, 190–91
Taste, 35
Telephone communication, 88, 118
Thayer, Lee, 187

Time, as form of nonverbal communication, 99
Tolman, Edward C., 143
Total system communication networks, 177
Touch, 35, 94, 96
Transmission, 16, 18
Trust, 77, 78, 132, 155

U

Uncertainty, 73
Understanding, 19

V

Values, 5, 55–61
Verbal communication, 16, 79–84, 118
  appropriateness, 84
  definition of, 78
  meaning, 79, 81
  style, 81–84
Visualization, 2
Vocal communication, 16, 18, 80, 84–89
  appropriateness, 87–89
  articulation and pronunciation, 85–87
  definition of, 78
  sound production, 85

W

Waiting room, 114, 115
Watzlawick, Paul, 29, 69
Wentz, Frank, 148
Wilmot, William, 206
Work roles, 65–66